New Insights into

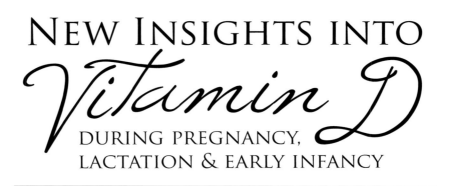

Vitamin D

During Pregnancy, Lactation & Early Infancy

Carol L. Wagner, M.D., with Sarah N. Taylor, M.D.
and Bruce W. Hollis, Ph.D.

Department of Pediatrics, Pediatric Nutritional Research Center,
Darby Children's Research Institute,
Medical University of South Carolina, Charleston, SC

NEW INSIGHTS INTO VITAMIN D DURING PREGNANCY,
LACTATION AND EARLY INFANCY

Hale Publishing, L.P.
Amarillo, TX 79106-7017
806-376-9900
800-378-1317
www.iBreastfeeding.com
www.Hale-Publishing.com

***

Address correspondence to:
Carol L. Wagner, M.D.
Medical University of SC
173 Ashley Avenue,   MSN 513
Charleston, SC 29425
Telephone #: (843) 792-8829
Fax #: (843) 792-7828
Email: wagnercl@musc.edu

Supported in part by grants from NIH 5 R01 HD047511, NIH 5 R01
HD043921, the Thrasher Research Fund, and from the General Clinical
Research Center/now CTRC, Medical University of South Carolina, Charleston,
SC, NIH #RR01070.

Disclosure: Bruce W. Hollis, Ph.D. serves as a scientific consultant for Diasorin
Inc., Minneapolis, Minnesota. Drs. Carol L. Wagner and Sarah N. Taylor have
nothing to disclose.

Library of Congress Control Number: 2010921902
ISBN-13: 978-0-9823379-6-7

Printed in Canada.

To the hundreds of women and children who have participated and continue to participate in our vitamin D studies; to our vitamin D research team without whose help our research would not be possible; to our children Cayden, Jefferson, James, Ian, Sarah, and Stephen; to our spouses for their understanding about our passion for studying vitamin D; and lastly, to our parents, who were there from the beginning.

TABLE OF CONTENTS

1. SUMMARY

Vitamin D is the substrate precursor to one of the most powerful hormones in the body--1,25-dihydroxy-vitamin D, which has profound effects on metabolism and immune function that extend far beyond the traditional thinking of bone and calcium metabolism. We are only just beginning to understand its effects on various organ systems throughout the body—from epidemiological studies to its actions at the cellular level. Vitamin D has been linked to inflammatory and long-latency diseases, such as multiple sclerosis, rheumatoid arthritis, lupus, tuberculosis, diabetes, cardiovascular disease, and various cancers, to name a few. How can such a simple "vitamin" be involved in such diverse groups of diseases? What is the mechanism? What does it mean to you as the individual, as the practitioner, or as the public policy maker?

In this book, we will review the history of vitamin D and its link with rickets, its discovery in the early twentieth century as the active component in cod liver oil that prevents rickets, and how changes in lifestyle have led to one of the largest epidemics of nutrient deficiency beginning in the late 20th century. We will review how our limited understanding about vitamin D set the stage for recommendations that unknowingly are now associated with states of vitamin D deficiency. We present the evolving understanding of vitamin D's function in the context of bone mineralization and development, but also in terms of its effect on immune function, and review how that understanding has influenced our views on vitamin D requirements. We will focus on the results of deficiency states during pregnancy and lactation, the implications of that deficiency during early childhood and later adult life, the controversies surrounding vitamin D supplementation, and what can be done by public health officials and healthcare professionals to prevent vitamin D deficiency today and in the future.

2. Introduction

There is a renewed interest in vitamin D today. With a rise in the prevalence of vitamin D deficiency in various populations across the globe, particularly in individuals of darker pigmentation or with limited access to sunlight, there has been an urgent need to understand why this has occurred and what effect such deficiency has across the lifespan.[1] Long-standing vitamin D deficiency is linked to a myriad of disease states through its putative effect on the immune system (Liu et al., 2006). It is only with large numbers of individuals who suffer from vitamin D deficiency that such connections between deficiency and disease could be discerned, and through modern laboratory techniques that the mechanisms delineated.

How did we get to this place—this place of widespread vitamin D deficiency? What is the evidence that we, in fact, have vitamin D deficiency at epidemic proportions in the U.S. and in other countries throughout the world? People ask on a daily basis—in their social circles, at the doctor's office, on call-in radio shows, on listservs and websites—is vitamin D *really* important? Or, is vitamin D the new vitamin E and vitamin C of the 21st century, the current fad "cure-all"? Health shows, magazine articles, and the lay press write reviews trying to decipher the plethora of emerging data that is published on a weekly basis about the benefits and potential dangers of vitamin D supplementation. The individual is inundated with a vast amount of information to decipher, and to ultimately decide, what should I do?

---

[1] (Acharya, Annamali, Taub, & Field, 2004; Bandeira et al., 2006; Chiu, Chu, Go, & Soad, 2004; Dawodu, Agarwal, Hossain, Kochiyil, & Zayed, 2003; Dawodu & Wagner, 2007; Ford, Ajani, McGuire, & Liu, 2005; Fuleihan et al., 2001; Fuleihan & Deeb, 1999; Holick, 2004; Hollis & Wagner, 2004b; Hypponen et al., 2004; Lehtonen-Veromaa, et al., 1999; Liu et al., 2005; Nesby-O'Dell et al., 2002; Olmez, Bober, Buyukgebiz, & Cimrin, 2006; Otani, Iwasaki, Sasazuki, Inoue, & Tsugane, 2007; Pettifor, 2005; Pittas et al., 2006; Plotnikoff & Quigley, 2003; Robien, Cutler, & Lazovich, 2007; Schleithoff et al., 2003; Schleithoff et al., 2006; Thomas et al., 1998; Tseng, Breslow, Graubard, & Ziegler, 2005; Ward, 2005; Wu et al., 2007; Ziegler, Hollis, Nelson, & Jeter, 2006; Zittermann, Schleithoff, & Koerfer, 2005, 2006, 2007; Zittermann et al., 2003; Acharya et al., 2004; Chiu et al., 2004; Holick, 2004; Hollis & Wagner, 2004; Hypponen et al., 2004; Ford et al., 2005; Liu et al., 2005; Pettifor, 2005; Tseng et al., 2005; Ward, 2005; Zittermann et al., 2005; Bandeira et al., 2006; Olmez et al., 2006; Pittas et al., 2006; Schleithoff et al., 2006; Ziegler et al., 2006; Zittermann et al., 2006; Dawodu & Wagner, 2007; Otani et al., 2007; Robien et al., 2007; Wu et al., 2007; Zittermann et al., 2007.)

If you are a pregnant or lactating woman, that question becomes even more important, as you are not deciding just for you, but for your unborn child, developing newborn, and infant. If you are a health care professional, you must weigh the evidence and decades-old concern that if you supplement a woman with more than 400 IU vitamin D per day, you will make her vitamin D toxic and her unborn fetus will be at risk for birth defects. Until recently, such was the view held by medical experts for decades. If you are a public health official, you are faced with the decision of recommending higher amounts of vitamin D in vitamins and revising the national recommendations of the upper limit of what is safe for various age groups, or erring on the side of caution in maintaining the *status quo* because it is what has happened for the last four decades, and it is "safe." There is always the underlying tenet of "Do no harm," which must be at the heart of every recommendation.

Given the issues and seeming confusion surrounding vitamin D, we recognize the need for a concise and up-to-date overview about vitamin D. This book serves this purpose. We have organized this book into twelve sections (including this one), with references at the end, that can be read in their entirety or individually with much cross-referencing to help you, the reader, find answers to your questions about vitamin D. The answers are a work in progress: as new information became known about vitamin D, recommendations have changed, but the story is unfolding, and the recommendations will continue to change with refinement of our understanding of vitamin D. Welcome to this exciting time in vitamin D research! Enjoy the journey as we travel back in time to gain perspective and fast forward to the 21st century.

3. THE TIMELINE OF VITAMIN D

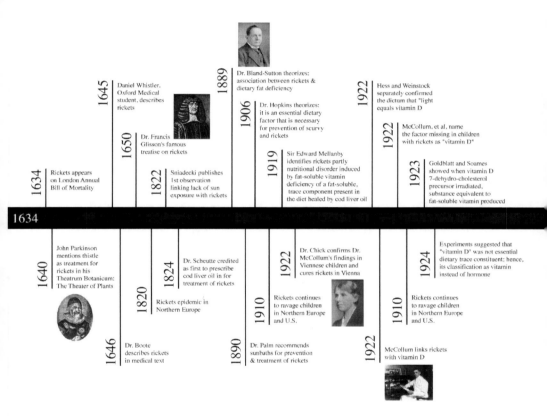

1645 Daniel Whistler, Oxford Medical student, describes rickets

1650 Dr. Francis Glisson's famous treatise on rickets

1889 Dr. Bland-Sutton theorizes: association between rickets & dietary fat deficiency

1906 Dr. Hopkins theorizes: it is an essential dietary factor that is necessary for prevention of scurvy and rickets

1919 Sir Edward Mellanby identifies rickets partly nutritional disorder induced by fat-soluble vitamin deficiency of a fat-soluble, trace component present in the diet healed by cod liver oil

1922 Hess and Weinstock separately confirmed the dictum that "light equals vitamin D

1922 McCollum, et al, name the factor missing in children with rickets as "vitamin D"

1923 Goldblatt and Soames showed when vitamin D 7-dehydro-cholesterol precursor irradiated, substance equivalent to fat-soluble vitamin produced

1634 Rickets appears on London Annual Bill of Mortality

1822 Sniadecki publishes 1st observation linking lack of sun exposure with rickets

1634

1640 John Parkinson mentions thistle as treatment for rickets in his Theatrum Botanicum: The Theater of Plants

1820 Rickets epidemic in Northern Europe

1824 Dr. Scheutte credited as first to prescribe cod liver oil in for treatment of rickets

1922 Dr. Chick confirms Dr. McCollum's findings in Viennese children and cures rickets in Vienna

1910 Rickets continues to ravage children in Northern Europe and U.S.

1924 Experiments suggested that "vitamin D" was not essential dietary trace constituent; hence, its classification as vitamin instead of hormone

1910 Rickets continues to ravage children in Northern Europe and U.S.

1646 Dr. Boote describes rickets in medical text

1890 Dr. Palm recommends sunbaths for prevention & treatment of rickets

1922 McCollum links rickets with vitamin D

11

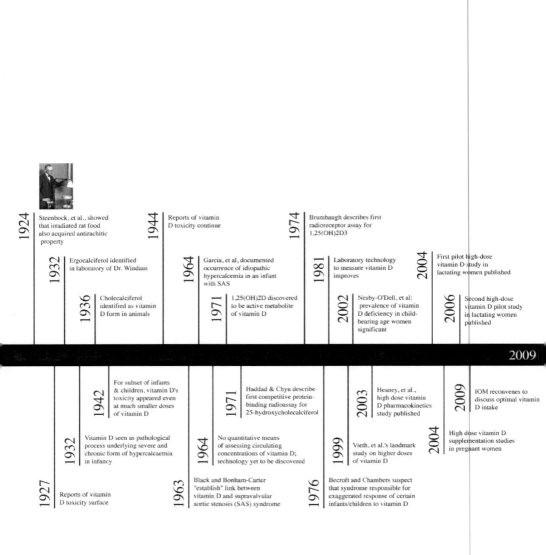

1924 Steenbock, et al., showed that irradiated rat food also acquired antirachitic property

1932 Ergocalciferol identified in laboratory of Dr. Windaus

1936 Cholecalciferol identified as vitamin D form in animals

1944 Reports of vitamin D toxicity continue

1964 Garcia, et al, documented occurrence of idiopathic hypercalcemia in an infant with SAS

1971 1,25(OH)2D discovered to be active metabolite of vitamin D

1974 Brumbaugh describes first radioreceptor assay for 1,25(OH)2D3

1981 Laboratory technology to measure vitamin D improves

2002 Nesby-O'Dell, et al: prevalence of vitamin D deficiency in child-bearing age women significant

2004 First pilot high-dose vitamin D study in lactating women published

2006 Second high-dose vitamin D pilot study in lactating women published

2009

1927 Reports of vitamin D toxicity surface

1932 Vitamin D seen as pathological process underlying severe and chronic form of hypercalcaemia in infancy

1942 For subset of infants & children, vitamin D's toxicity appeared even at much smaller doses of vitamin D

1963 Black and Bonham-Carter "establish" link between vitamin D and supravalvular aortic stenosis (SAS) syndrome

1964 No quantitative means of assessing circulating concentrations of vitamin D; technology yet to be discovered

1971 Haddad & Chyu describe first competitive protein-binding radioassay for 25-hydroxycholecalciferol

1976 Becroft and Chambers suspect that syndrome responsible for exaggerated response of certain infants/children to vitamin D

1999 Vieth, et al.'s landmark study on higher doses of vitamin D

2003 Heaney, et al., high dose vitamin D pharmacokinetics study published

2004 High dose vitamin D supplementation studies in pregnant women

2009 IOM reconvenes to discuss optimal vitamin D intake

4. The History of Rickets and the Discovery of Vitamin D

"It is but little realized how great and how widespread is the part played by rickets in civilized communities. If the matter ended with bony deformities obvious to the eye it would be bad enough, but investigations have demonstrated that such deformities only represent a small part of the cases affected." Sir Edward Mellanby, 1919, "An Experimental Investigation of Rickets," published in The Lancet, volume 1, page 407.

In any review about vitamin D, there must be mention of rickets, as their histories are interwoven. Our early understanding about vitamin D's role in health comes from our study of patients with rickets. What is rickets?

Rickets

The most obvious aspect of rickets is its incurred physical deformities. Children with rickets, then and now, could be identified by deformities of the skeleton, including enlargement of the head, joints of the long bones, and rib cage ("rachitic rosary"—both palpable and seen on radiograph), curvature of the spine and thighs, coupled with generalized muscle weakness, lethargy, and a higher risk of infection (Park, 1923; Hess, 1929; Weick, 1967; Rehman, 1994).

The great French physician Armand Trousseau wrote in 1868:

> *Rickets is a disease of early infancy: it generally supervenes at the apoch of dentition, that is to say, toward the end of the first year of life, or during the first six months of the second year...the lesions which it has produced often remain and are incurable, continuing in life, so that the unfortunate sufferers retain horrible deformities...due to softening of the bones: so great is the softening, that when one tries to bend the limbs in their continuity, very great flexion is the result...while the cavity of the true pelvis is contracted,*

the large pelvis has, on the contrary, a greater capacity…the greater pelvis
becomes spread out, and this spreading out contributes to the contraction of
the lesser pelvis (translated by Sir Cormack, London: New Sydenham Society,
1872, excerpt from Dunn, 1999).

He aptly demonstrated what came to be called the "Trousseau sign"[2] that resulted from severe hypocalcemia associated with severe vitamin D deficiency (Chick, 1976). Also known as "the English disease," Dr. Chick wrote:

[Rickets is]…caused by a failure of the cartilage to calcify in the joints of
children so that they lack stability and bend under the weight of the body.
The spine becomes curved, the leg bones are bent and there is swelling around
the joints. In severe cases deformities may occur which will last for a lifetime
(Chick, 1976, p. 43).

The observations of these great physicians remain valid today. What has changed is our understanding of the metabolism and pathophysiology of rickets and its underlying causes, not the least of which is vitamin D.

The morbidity and mortality associated with rickets were not insignificant. According to Dr. O'Riordan at the University College of London, what appears to be the first written mention of rickets and the first mortality report of the disease was the Annual Bill of Mortality for the City of London: in 1634, of the 10,900 deaths, 14 were attributed to rickets (O'Riordan, 2006). Twenty-five years later, in 1659, there were 441 recorded entries of deaths attributed to rickets (O'Riordan, 2006). It is likely that while the true incidence of the disease may have increased, concurrently, the diagnosis of the disease made by physicians and knowledge of the disease by the general public had increased as well.

---

[2] Trousseau sign is a sign of latent tetany due to hypocalcemia. To elicit the sign, one uses a cuff, such as a blood pressure cuff, placed around the arm and inflated to a pressure greater than the systolic blood pressure, held in place for 3 minutes, thereby occluding the brachial artery. In the absence of blood flow, the patient will have spasm of the muscles of the hand and forearm. This is due to the patient's state of hypocalcemia and resulting neuromuscular irritability. Specifically, the wrist and metacarpophalangeal joints flex, the distal interphalangeal (DIP) and proximal interphalangeal (PIP) joints extend, and the fingers adduct. The sign also is known as main d'accoucheur (French for "hand of the obstetrician") as the spasm induced resembles the position of an obstetrician's hand in delivering a baby. Trousseau, A. (1872). Lectures on Clinical Medicine, Delivered at the Hotel Dieu. Translated by Sir John Cormack. London: New Sydenham Society.

Later, in 1877 in the U.S., Senator (1877) reported that 25% of all Philadelphia children under age five were rachitic. In the United States alone between 1910-1961, 13,807 deaths were attributed to rickets, of which 8,397 involved infants less than 12 months (Weick, 1967). Rickets was viewed, even then, as a major health problem for young children. It appeared with increasing regularity as people began their exodus from rural farming communities to urban areas, which—in turn, brought about lifestyle and environmental changes that limited sunlight exposure (Park, 1923; Hess, 1929; Mozolowski, 1939; O'Riordan, 2006).

Rickets is an example of extreme vitamin D deficiency, with a peak incidence between 3 and 18 months of age. A state of deficiency occurs typically weeks to months before rickets is obvious on physical examination. It is important to remember that the deficiency state may also present with hypocalcemic seizures (Binet & Kooh, 1996; Ladhani, Srinivasan, Buchanan, & Allgrove, 2004; Hatun et al., 2005), growth failure, lethargy, irritability, and a predisposition to respiratory infections during infancy (Stearns & Jeans, 1936; Molgaard & Michaelsen, 2003; Ladhani et al., 2004; Najada, Habashneh, & Khader, 2004; Pawley & Bishop 2004). Najada et al. (2004), in their retrospective analysis of children presenting with vitamin D deficiency in the United Kingdom, found two types of presentations: (1) symptomatic hypocalcemia (including seizures), occurring during periods of rapid growth, with increased metabolic demands, long before any physical findings or radiologic evidence of vitamin D deficiency occurred; and (2) a more chronic disease state, with rickets and/or decreased bone mineralization and either normocalcemia or asymptomatic hypocalcemia.[3]

As we discuss in more detail later in **Sections 6-9**, rickets occurs due to diminished absorption of dietary calcium and the mineral phosphorus that is a direct consequence of inadequate levels of $1,25(OH)_2D$ in the blood. Without calcium and phosphorus, the body cannot build strong bones; hence, the formation of rickets in children and osteoporosis in older individuals. The lack of vitamin D goes well beyond bone and affects other processes within the body, which helps to explain the observations of associated disease states with rickets and osteoporosis.

---

[3] For a more complete review of nutritional rickets and its management, please refer to the Lawson Wilkins Pediatric Endocrine Society recent publication on the topic: Misra et al., 2008. "Vitamin D deficiency in children and its management: review of current knowledge and recommendations." Pediatrics 122(2): 398-417.

History and its tendency to repeat itself—those issues continue to exist today (Nesby-O'Dell et al., 2002). Rickets was and continues to be a disease that has a significant effect on the developing child and that child's well-being. It is not surprising, then, that attempts were made, even in antiquity, to better understand the disease and its causes.

Along the Timeline of Vitamin D's History

Long before the industrial revolution, ancient records as far back as Homer in 900 BC and the 1st century AD make reference to children afflicted with "Genus IV" and "gibbosus or cyrtosis," meaning curve (Hess, 1929; Weick, 1967). Soranus Ephesius, 130 AD, a Roman physician of that era, wrote about bony deformities that were observed more frequently in infants who lived in Rome and Greece, which he attributed to lack of nurture and hygiene by Roman mothers (Hess, 1929). Galen, who lived during this time as well, described the classic bony deformities of rickets (Hess, 1929). Deformities that affected the spine were called rhachitis, from "rhacia" or spine (Weick, 1967). Whether or not this was true rickets remains to be proved, but it is likely that in areas of the world with little sunlight or with lack of sunlight exposure and lack of marine animals as a source of vitamin D, there were children afflicted with the disease who had "rickets."

Scientific writings about "the rickets" did not occur, however, until the mid 17th century. In his review of rickets, Dr. O'Riordan (2006) makes note of two important points: While reports of deaths due to rickets appeared as early as 1634 in the Annual Bill of Mortality for the City of London, it was not mentioned in a medical text until 1640, when John Parkinson published his works *Theatrum Botanicum: The Theater of Plants* and mentions the use of common thistle in the treatment of "the rickets." The first true scientific report on rickets, however, does not appear until 1645, when an Oxford medical student by the name of Daniel Whistler first described the disease, which was rampant where he lived in southwest England, in his thesis that he presented to the University of Leiden (Ruhrah, 1925; Hess, 1929; Still, 1931; Chick, 1976; O'Riordan, 2006). Another general medical book published by Dr. Boote in 1646 mentions rickets in Chapter Twelve (O'Riordan, 2006). This was followed by anatomist Dr. Francis Glissen's more scientific treatise (coauthored by Bate and Regemorter) about rickets in 1650, which remains a classic historic resource on the disease (Glissen, 1650; Glissen, 1668; Ruhrah, 1925; Hess, 1929; O'Riordan, 2006). Despite these observations, the following two centuries led to little advancement in the understanding or treatment of rickets (Rajakumar, 2003). There were numerous health regimens and concoctions, including herbal remedies, that were espoused to cure "rickets" (Weick, 1967).

The incidence of rickets escalated from the early reports in London in the 17th century to its peak in the 19th century during the industrial revolution. By the early 1800's, rickets was an epidemic in northern Europe and in industrialized northern regions of the United States. In 1822, Sniadecki published the first observation, which linked the lack of sun exposure with rickets (Mozolowski, 1939). He found that children who lived in cities in Poland had a higher incidence of rickets compared with children from the countryside who were disease-free. Dr. Scheutte is credited as being the first to prescribe cod liver oil in 1824 for the treatment of rickets (Guy, 1923; McCollum, 1957). Without knowing why it worked, fish liver oils—particularly cod liver oil—were used to treat rickets (Hess, 1929). It would take another 100 years before the specific agent in cod liver oil, namely vitamin D, would be identified.

The importance of sunlight and cod liver oil in preventing rickets gradually became more widely accepted. As evidenced by the writings of Palm and others, there was recognition of the role of sunlight in the development of rickets, with reports of lack of sunlight and poor diet leading to "the rickets" (Rajakumar, 2003). In 1890, Palm noted that despite a superior diet and sanitary living conditions, infants living in Britain had an increased incidence of rickets when compared to infants living in the tropics. He then recommended sun-baths for the prevention and treatment of rickets (Palm, 1890). The year before, Dr. Bland-Sutton theorized that there was an association between rickets and a dietary fat deficiency (Rajakumar, 2003; Rajakumar & Thomas, 2005; Chesney & Hedberg, 2009). He observed florid rickets in lion cubs at the London Zoo who subsisted on a diet of boneless lean meat, which he could reverse with the addition of cod liver oil and crushed bones. It was Dr. Hopkins who further theorized in 1906 that it was an essential dietary factor that was necessary for the prevention of such diseases as scurvy and rickets (Hopkins, 1906).

Two lines of thought were emerging—that lack of sunlight was at the root of the disease, while others believed that it was a dietary factor, such as that found in cod liver oil, which could prevent the disease. Interestingly, both points of view were actually correct. Scientists were closer to "a truth" about vitamin D; however, definitive proof that either path—diet or sunlight—was an integral part of the rickets prevention equation would not come for another twenty years.

The Age of Nutritional Sciences and the Discovery of Vitamin D

Despite advances in the understanding of the root cause of rickets, at the start of the 20th century, rickets was still an epidemic in the northern, industrialized regions of the United States and Europe, with 96% of infants demonstrating microscopic findings of the disease at autopsy (Hess, 1922; Rajakumar, 2003). Perhaps it was the persistence of the epidemic that served as an impetus to understand the disease, but the major breakthroughs in our understanding about the causative factors of rickets did not occur until the period of 1910-1930. It was during this time that nutrition as an experimental science and the appreciation of the existence of vitamins, and in the case of vitamin D, hormones were realized.

Testing his premise that a fat-soluble dietary factor for health prevented rickets, Sir Edward Mellanby conducted the first experiments designed to find the underlying cause and effect, and thus, possible treatment of rickets (Mellanby & Cantag, 1919). His experiments involved dogs that were raised exclusively indoors (in the absence of sunlight or ultraviolet light). Using an *in vivo* dog model, Mellanby devised a diet of low-fat milk and bread to unequivocally establish that the bone disease—rickets— was, at least in part, a nutritional disorder and could be induced by a deficiency of a fat-soluble, trace component present in the diet that could be healed consistently with the administration of cod liver oil. In 1921 Mellanby wrote:

> *The action of fats in rickets is due to a vitamine or accessory food factor which they contain, probably identical with the Fat-soluble vitamine (p. 82).*

Furthermore, he established that cod liver oil was an excellent antirachitic agent (Mellanby, 1921). He also noted earlier that if "…the matter ended with bony deformities obvious to the eye it would be bad enough, but investigations have demonstrated that such deformities represent only a small part of the cases affected," and that the "...rachitic child, in fact, carries the stigma of the disease throughout life in the form of defective teeth (Mellanby & Cantag, 1919, p. 407). More amazing today were Mellanby's observations in 1919 that the rachitic child was at risk for other associated conditions or diseases:

> Nor is this the most serious part of the evil, for the reduced resistance to other diseases of the rachitic child and animal is so marked that the causative factor of rickets may be the secret of immunity and non-immunity to many of the children's diseases which result in the high death-rate associated with urban conditions. It is a striking fact to remember that in the West of Ireland, where the death rate is only 30 per 1000, rickets is an unknown disease, whereas in poor urban districts of this country where rickets is rife the death-rate in children varies from 100 to 300 per 1000 (p. 407).

His findings were confirmed in puppies fed rickets-producing diets and "...by other workers in rats, children, and dogs; it cleared up quickly, if caught at an early stage, on the addition of cod-liver oil to the diet." There were four broad categories of diseases in the rachitic animals that were noted by Mellanby: (1) heart failure during anesthesia and a prolonged recovery with anorexia and weight loss; (2) several types of nervous defects that included incoordination, paralysis, convulsions and tetany [what we know today is caused by critically low levels of calcium in the body]; (3) keratomalacia; and (4) "...increased susceptibility and lowered resistance to distemper and other catarrhal conditions, broncho-pneumonia, and skin affections like mange." Beginning in the late 20th century, these associations continue to be "rediscovered" as manifestations of human diseases (Holick, Perez, & Raab, 1992; Brunvand, Haga, Tangsrud, & Haug, 1995; Munger, Levin, Hollis, Howard, & Ascherio, 2006; Schleithoff et al., 2006; Zittermann, Schleithoff, & Koerfer, 2006; Laaksi et al., 2007; Roth, Jones, Prosser, Robinson, & Vohra, 2009).

Concurrent with the work of Mellanby, Dr. E.V. McCollum and his associates at Johns Hopkins University expanded on the earlier thinking of Hopkins (1906). They determined that the nutritional factor deficient in diets leading to rickets was a substance they called "vitamin D" (Shipley, Park, McCollum, Simmonds, & Parsons, 1921; McCollum, Simmonds, Becket, & Shipley, 1922; Guy, 1923;

Park, 1923; McCollum, 1957; McCollum, 1964; DeLuca, 1988). By bubbling oxygen through a preparation of the "fat-soluble vitamin," they were able to distinguish between vitamin A (which was inactivated) and vitamin D (which retained activity). They also were able to produce a model of rickets in rats fed purified diets containing an unfavorable balance of calcium and phosphorus, which could be prevented if certain fats were added to the diet (McCollum et al., 1922; McCollum, 1964). Clinical confirmation of these findings came from Dr. Hariette Chick and her colleagues in 1922: when working with post-World War I malnourished Viennese children who had a high prevalence of rickets, she was able to cure the children on diets of either whole milk or cod liver oil (Chick, 1976; Wolf, 2004).

While dietary manipulations could prevent, resolve or exacerbate rickets, there were scientists who pursued the sunlight/ultraviolet light theory of rickets. In the same year that Mellanby was studying rachitic puppies and diet, Dr. K. Huldschinsky in Germany showed conclusive evidence via x-ray changes that when children with rickets were repeatedly exposed to mercury vapor quartz lamp rays (i.e., ultraviolet light), healing of the rachitic process ensued (Kramer et al., 1922). In 1921, Hess and Unger showed that sunlight exposure of at least 30 minutes per day up to several hours could cure infantile rickets (Hess & Unger, 1921a). They further showed that "…infants born about the beginning of February were least likely to develop rickets; they are subjected to only a few months of lack of sunlight and then enjoy a prolonged period of intense sunlight" (Hess & Unger, 1921b; Hess & Unger, 1922a).

In 1923, Goldblatt and Soames identified that when the precursor of vitamin D 7-dehydro-cholesterol found in the epidermis of the skin was irradiated with sunlight or ultraviolet light, a substance equivalent to the fat-soluble vitamin was produced (Goldblatt & Soames, 1923). Hess and Weinstock confirmed the dictum that "light equals vitamin D" (Hess, 1922; Hess & Weinstock, 1923). In their experiments, Hess and Weinstock excised a small portion of skin that was irradiated with ultraviolet light, and then fed it to groups of rachitic rats. The skin that had been irradiated provided an absolute protection against rickets, whereas the unirradiated skin provided no protection whatsoever. It was clear from these experiments that these animals were able to produce adequate quantities of the "fat-soluble vitamin." In parallel studies to the work of Hess and Weinstock (Hess, Unger et al., 1922b, c), Steenbock and Nelson (Steenbock, 1924; Steenbock & Nelson, 1924) and Steenbock and Black (1924) found that rat food, which was irradiated with ultraviolet light, also acquired the property of being antirachitic.

The dietary experiments suggested to the scientists of the day that "vitamin D" belonged to the class of organic substances occurring in foods called "vitamins " that was essential to the nutrition and normal metabolic functioning of the body. Despite studies that demonstrated the skin's ability to synthesize vitamin D from its precursor following sunlight exposure, diet was considered the main source of vitamin D, a view that plagues us to this day.[4]

Additional understanding about vitamin D and its role in maintaining health came from the published work of Park (1923) and the ongoing work of Harriette Chick and her coworkers (Chick, 1976) who were able to confirm independently the use of cod liver oil (vitamin D) supplementation and sun exposure for the prevention and treatment of rickets. They also noted the seasonality of rickets, "which was in accordance with the wide experiences of clinicians that rickets developed in winter and spring and healed in summer" (Chick, 1976). By the 1930s, routine vitamin D supplementation, sun exposure, and milk fortification in the United States almost led to the eradication of rickets (Park, 1923; Park, 1940).

The Chemical Structures of Vitamin D

The chemical structures of vitamin D were first delineated in the 1930s by Dr. Windaus at the University of Göttingen in Germany (Windaus, Linsert, Littringhaus, & Weidlinch, 1932). Vitamin D_2 or ergocalciferol, which could be produced by ultraviolet irradiation of ergosterol, was chemically characterized in 1932. It took another 4 years for vitamin D_3 (cholecalciferol) to be chemically characterized. Vitamin D_3 was synthesized following ultraviolet irradiation of 7-dehydrocholesterol. Breakthroughs in laboratory technology and a better understanding of chemistry and the concept of chemical pathways came about,

---

[4] The significance of this—that vitamin D was deemed a "vitamin" and not the substrate precursor to the active hormone—would impact millions of individuals throughout the world by the end of the twentieth century. It had everything to do with our expectation that a well-balanced diet and occasional sun exposure could provide all that one needed and set the stage for one of the largest nutritional epidemics in history.

which allowed enhanced isolation and identification of compounds. Virtually simultaneously, the elusive antirachitic (or anti-rickets) component of cod liver oil was shown to be identical to the newly characterized vitamin D_3. Today, we know that the form produced by all animals is, in fact, cholecalciferol or vitamin D_3, while that synthesized by plants is ergocalciferol or vitamin D_2. The collective scientific inquiries and findings of scientists of that time clearly established that the antirachitic substance vitamin D was chemically a steroid, more specifically, a **secosteroid** (Brockmann, 1936; Crowfoot-Hodgkin, Webster, & Dunitz, 1957).

While there were advances in laboratory techniques to isolate vitamin D and trace its metabolism and metabolic processes, there were no reliable measures that could be utilized easily and consistently in the clinics and at the bedside. There was an exuberance of prescribing vitamins—sometimes at pharmacological doses that led to reports of toxicity in the post-World War II era in Great Britain. Vitamin D went from being the "darling of vitamins" to being viewed as a potential toxin, especially to pregnant women (Leake, 1936; Blumberg, Forbes, & Fraser, 1963; Friedman & Roberts, 1966). The "Dangers of Vitamin D" became more of a concern and dominated the field of vitamin D research for the next 40 years (American Academy of Pediatrics, Committee on Nutrition, 1963).

5. THE DANGERS OF VITAMIN D

As early as the 1920's, reports of vitamin D toxicity surfaced (Pfannenstiel, 1927; Kreitmair & Moll, 1928; Harris & Innes, 1931). In an era when individual levels were not easily and reliably measured to document "deficiency" or "sufficiency," individuals were prescribed or given hundreds of thousands of IU's of vitamin D. This resulted in the classic symptomatology of toxicity or hypercalcemia within weeks or months through the actions of the active form of vitamin D—$1,25(OH)_2D$, acting independently from parathyroid hormone, which is suppressed.[5] As Dr. Reinhold Vieth states in a recent review (Vieth, 2009b, p. 441):

> *Any agent that can elicit a biological effect will be harmful if the amount taken is sufficiently high....High concentrations of vitamin D are toxic to rats and have been used to poison them (40,000 IU can kill a rat, which is equivalent on a weight basis, of approximately 7-10 million IU in a 70-kg human)...*

There is no question that there can be toxicity associated with vitamin D taken orally. Harris, Moore, Innes, Ham, Lewis and others reported that hypervitaminosis D was a real and reproducible entity that could be replicated in the laboratory using rat and rabbit models (Harris & Moore, 1928; Harris & Innes, 1931; Ham & Lewis, 1934). The investigators gave pharmacological doses to rats, which was similar to the amounts prescribed or given to some children and adults (Harris & Innes, 1931). Since that time, reports of vitamin D toxicity have occurred—in each case involving ingestion of hundreds of thousands of international units of

---

[5] $1,25(OH)_2D$ promotes hypercalcemia by a number of different mechanisms that include: (1) enhanced absorption of calcium and phosphorus from the small intestine; (2) enhanced bone mineralization, especially at the growth plate; and (3) enhanced calcium reabsorption in the distal tubules of the kidney. Hypercalcemia, whatever its cause, leads to decreased conduction in nerve and muscle, and there is associated anorexia, nausea/vomiting, weakness, fatigue, lassitude, polyuria/polydipsia and nocturia. Laboratory parameter will confirm one's suspicion of hypercalcemia and the involvement of other organ systems, such as the kidney, with acute and/or chronic renal failure, and variable degrees of hyperphosphatemia (Chick, 1976; Jacobus et al., 1992; Misra et al., 2008; Leake, 1936; Howard & Meyer, 1948; Davies, 2009; Allgrove, 2009). Excessive calcification of the epiphysis, as well as metaphysis and extramedullary calcifications that are detected clinically, can be confirmed by radiographs (Howard & Meyer, 1948:. DeWind, 1961).

vitamin D taken for weeks to months (DeWind, 1961; Down, Polak, & Regan, 1979; Jacobus et al., 1992). In 1948, Debré wrote about the dosage that causes such toxicity and death (Debre, 1948, p. 790):

> *What are signs by which one can make a prognosis? The total dosage of the drug is not the main factor. However, it is true that the children who died (at age of 20 and 16 months) had received, respectively, 11,200,000 and 18,200,000 units. The mild cases occurred when only 3,000,000 to 6,000,000 units had been given.* [6]

Clearly, these children were given pharmacological doses of vitamin D and not doses within the physiological range.

Debré, in his careful study of 21 patients who presented with vitamin D toxicity, noted that the first symptom was significant and abrupt onset of anorexia, which was present in all the cases. There was often nausea and vomiting, which would occur days later with sudden onset. In addition, his patients would describe severe thirst (polydipsia) and associated polyuria. Skeletal bony and muscular pain and cramps could also occur.[7] Laboratory parameters included elevated serum calcium levels above 12 and progressive rise of blood urea nitrogen, all symptoms of hypercalcemia. With all of these observations, however, it was not possible to measure circulating 25(OH)D or vitamin D levels, so the diagnosis was made by clinical history and the supporting laboratory data as mentioned.

Similar results were reported by Dowling, Gauvain, and Macrae on the work of Dr. Dawson (Dowling, Gauvain, & Macrae, 1948, p. 432):

> *A valuable contribution to the study of toxicity was given by J. Dawson last July at Leeds. The material consisted of 186 cases (158 lupus, 28 other cases): of these, 34.7% showed a biochemical disturbance without clinical toxicity-that is, a rise in serum calcium to over 12 mg per 100 ml. or a diffusible calcium rise to over 7 mg. Of the 186 cases, 30 (16.2%) developed clinical*

---

[6] The dose that was prescribed to these children was at least 100,000 times greater than the dose prescribed to neonates today, and 10,000 times greater than the general upper limit given to adults.

[7] There is neuromuscular impairment that is directly related to the state of hypercalcemia. The elevation of calcium itself in the blood acts like a diuretic (hence the polyuria) by inhibiting antidiuretic hormone or vasopressin; this process in turn causes dehydration and renal impairment through diminished vascular kidney perfusion (Robinson et al., 1983;. Vieth, Pinto, et al., 2002). Mental confusion and lethargy were also notable.

toxicity, the onset of symptoms taking place at the mean dose of 16,400,000 I.U. Among the clinically toxic cases, the blood urea nitrogen was raised above 25 mg in all except four cases, and in these there was a rise from previous levels.

What made it more difficult to discern about vitamin D's safety was that for a subset of infants and children, vitamin D's toxicity appeared even at much smaller doses of vitamin D (Hild, 1942; Schlesinger, Butler, & Black, 1956; Daeschner & Daeschner, 1957). In addition, when given to pregnant women, there were reports of affected offspring with a specific constellation of findings (Schlesinger et al., 1956; Coleman, 1965). Through the work of several scientists between 1932 and 1953 (Lightwood, 1932; Anderson & Schlesinger, 1940; Lightwood & Payne, 1952; Schlesinger et al., 1956; Baggenstoss & Keith, 1941; Fanconi, Giradet, Schlesinger, Butler, & Black, 1952; Creery, 1953), the entity of idiopathic hypercalcemia of childhood was discovered and redefined. Russell and Young presented two cases of idiopathic hypercalcemia of infancy to the Royal Society of Medicine in 1954 with the following conclusion:

> *It may be concluded that the pathological process underlying the severe and chronic form of hypercalcaemia in infancy is intoxication with vitamin D or with some factor resembling its effects, probably initiated prenatally. …are likely due to the same causative factor operating later or with less intensity than in the cases with manifest skeletal changes and gross mental and physical retardation (Russell & Young, 1954, p. 1039-1040).*

With careful, meticulous study, definitive "proof" of vitamin D's toxicity and teratogenicity surfaced in the early 1960s. In 1963, Black and Bonham-Carter recognized that elfin facies observed in patients with severe idiopathic infantile hypercalcemia resembled peculiar facies observed in patients with supravalvular aortic stenosis (SAS) syndrome (Black & Bonham-Carter, 1963). Shortly thereafter, Garcia et al. documented the occurrence of idiopathic hypercalcemia in an infant with SAS. The infant also had peripheral pulmonary stenosis, mental retardation, elfin facies, and an elevated blood concentration of vitamin D (Garcia, Friedman, Kaback, & Rowe, 1964). Additional support came from the work of Friedman, Kaback, and Rowe (Friedman & Roberts, 1966).

Let's look at the issues surrounding vitamin D toxicity from another angle—that of the basic scientific understanding about vitamin D metabolism and technology necessary to accurately measure vitamin D during this time period. You may find it interesting that in 1964, there were no quantitative means of assessing circulating concentrations of vitamin D (Hollis, 1983). In fact, at that time, it was unproven that vitamin D was further metabolized within the body. Despite these limitations in scientific knowledge and technical capabilities, by 1967, vitamin D was viewed by many in the medical community as the cause of SAS syndrome (Taussig, 1966; Friedman, 1967; Friedman & Mills, 1967, 1969). Specifically, it was thought that maternal vitamin D supplementation during pregnancy and its associated toxicity caused SAS syndrome in a subgroup of susceptible fetuses and infants, resulting in the constellation of findings that included the elfin facies and other described findings. Animal models were developed to show that toxic excesses of vitamin D during pregnancy would result in SAS (Antia et al., 1967; Seelig, 1969). In those studies, pharmacologic doses—not physiologic doses— of vitamin D were given to animals, creating hypervitaminosis D with hypercalcemia. It is true that pharmacologic doses of vitamin D can lead to calcification of the aortic valve.

Several observations were made, many of which were accurate, but the etiology attributed to those observations was incorrect. Further investigation led researchers to find that the root cause of SAS in those individuals was not too much vitamin D *per se*, but a part of the spectrum of the genetic disorder called Williams Syndrome (Aravena et al., 2002). Williams Syndrome is a severe genetic affliction related to elastin gene disruption caused by deletion of elastin and contiguous genes on chromosome 7g11.23. The syndrome is characterized by multiorgan involvement (including SAS), dysmorphic facial features, and a distinctive cognitive profile (Morris & Mervis, 2000). Williams Syndrome patients often exhibit abnormal vitamin D metabolism, with an exaggerated increase in circulating 25(OH)D to orally administered vitamin D—*even doses as low as 400 IU* and, therefore, such patients are susceptible to bouts of idiopathic hypercalcemia. This relationship was suspected as early as 1976 (Becroft & Chambers, 1976), but was not definitively made until 1991 (Morris & Mervis, 2000).

As mentioned earlier, those cases of vitamin D toxicity that have occurred in infants, children, and adults without Williams Syndrome occurred when excessive doses (well in excess of 10,000 IU/day) were given. A recent case of vitamin D overdose confirms this premise: a 2 year old boy was erroneously given an entire ampule per day containing 600,000 IU instead of 2 drops per day and received a total of 2,400,000 IU in 4 days. This led to the characteristic toxicity of hypervitaminosis D from hypercalcemia (Barrueto, Wang-Flores, Howland, Hoffman, & Nelson, 2005).

Despite the enhanced understanding about the cause of supravalvular aortic stenosis in patients with Williams Syndrome, it was not known until recently what doses of vitamin D were physiologic and what were pharmacologic. Because of this lack of understanding, fear of causing hypervitaminosis D in individuals, particularly pregnant women, has continued to present (Hollis & Wagner, 2004a; Kleinman, 2009) This prompted the American Academy of Pediatrics to issue a statement about the use of vitamin D and its potential dangers in 1963.

From the 1960s on, there was a rapid decline of rickets, and many believed that modern medicine and science had "cured" rickets (Harrison, 1996). Unfortunately, nutritional rickets reemerged in the 1980s, particularly among African American and other darkly pigmented populations. The recurring characteristics of the reported cases were young age—particularly infants— darker pigmentation, often living at higher latitudes, and exclusive breastfeeding without vitamin D supplementation beyond 6 months of age (Rajakumar & Thomas, 2005). This finding led to a revised American Academy of Pediatrics (AAP) statement in 2003, recommending 200 IU per day of vitamin D supplementation to all infants receiving less than 500 ml of fortified formula per day to begin within the first 2 months of life (Gartner, Greer, et al., 2003). Continued reports of rickets, limited dietary sources of vitamin D, inadequate sun exposure for vitamin D synthesis, and an enhanced understanding of vitamin D physiology and its actions have led to the most recent revision of the AAP statement in 2008 (Wagner, Greer, & American Academy of Pediatrics, 2008). The current recommendations are for all infants and children to be supplemented with a minimum of 400 IU per day of vitamin D, beginning in the first few days of life (Wagner, Greer, et al., 2008). (See **Section 11** for further discussion on the topic.)

A wonderful review by Dr. Reinhold Vieth highlights the potential risks of additional vitamin D (Vieth, 2009b) and is well worth reading, as it clearly delineates how hypervitaminosis and hypercalcemia can occur. The issue today, however, is not too much vitamin D, but rather too little:

> *It is very unlikely that anyone following current advice regarding protection of the skin from solar ultraviolet (2) could achieve a serum 25(OH)D concentration greater than 75 nmol/L (30 ng/mL) without taking a vitamin D supplement (p. 441).*

In the past, the margin of safety of vitamin D was narrow, and as we discussed earlier, there was an understandable reluctance to recommend supplementation for fear of causing toxicity. With careful study, it appears that daily vitamin D dosing of less 10,000 IU/day for extended periods is safe. In this regard, Dr. Vieth wrote (Vieth, 2009b, p. 443):

> *Amounts of vitamin D much greater than physiologic levels, specifically greater than 10,000 IU per day, eventually become toxic once they occupy a meaningful proportion of circulating vitamin D-binding protein (DBP). High circulating concentrations of vitamin D metabolites displace $1,25(OH)_2D$ into the unbound, free phase that enters target tissues…*

This phenomenon of toxicity does not occur with doses of 4,000 IU vitamin D/day in an adult; at this dose, an individual achieves a circulating 25(OH)D level that is in the physiologic range, with adequate substrate to ensure adequate conversion of $1,25(OH)_2D$, not only by the kidneys, but by extrarenal tissue and cells as well. We and others have found that this daily intake of oral vitamin D is the amount that is comparable to what we as humans make with natural sun exposure, which is "far below the concentration required to cause physiochemical displacement of metabolites from vitamin DBP" (Vieth, 1990; Vieth, 2009b).

6. VITAMIN D STRUCTURE, NOMENCLATURE, AND SYNTHESIS

BY BRUCE W. HOLLIS, PH.D. AND CAROL L. WAGNER, M.D.

To understand vitamin D's function, a word must be said about its structure. Structure begets function. In reviewing the metabolism of vitamin D, you will come to appreciate its structure. As we begin this section, take a moment to look at this schematic of vitamin D that is found in **Figure 1**.

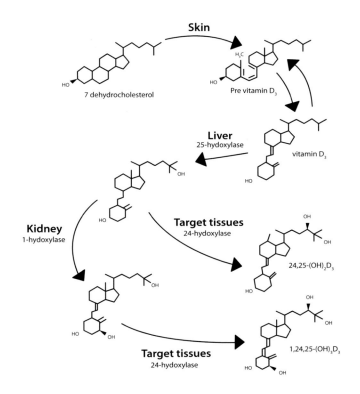

Figure 1. Vitamin D Structure

(2010, Christian Bressler)

As shown in **Figure 1**, there are two forms of Vitamin D: D_2 - ergocalciferol, synthesized by plants, and D_3 - cholecalciferol, synthesized by mammals. The major source for humans, vitamin D_3, is synthesized in the epidermis of the skin at UVB ranges 290-315nm (**Figure 2**).

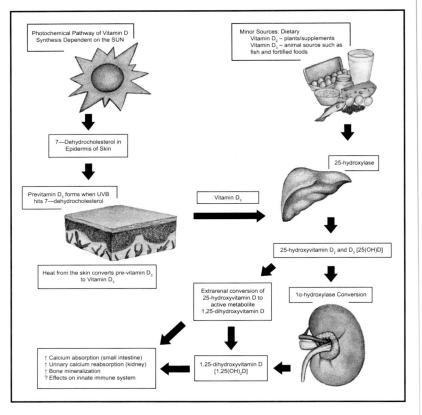

Figure 2. Synthesis of Major Sources of Vitamin D

(2010, Christian Bressler)

The UVB light in the range of 290-315 nm breaks the B-ring of 7-dehydrocholesterol to create previtamin D_3. Heat in the skin further isomerizes or transforms previtamin D_3 to vitamin D_3, which can then bind to the vitamin D binding protein. It is this second process—that of a light-induced conformational change of previtamin D to vitamin D_3— that allows the body to make endogenous vitamin D_3 following sunlight exposure (Esvelt, Schnoes, & Deluca, 1978).

From the epidermis or upper skin layer, the vitamin D_3 is transported to the liver, where it is converted to 25-hydroxyvitamin D (25(OH)D) by the enzyme 25-hydroxylase. *25(OH)D serves as the nutritional marker of vitamin D status, but it is not the active metabolite.* In order to become the active metabolite, 25(OH) D must be further hydroxylated in the kidney and other tissues to its active metabolite, 1, 25-dihydroxyvitamin D (1, 25(OH)$_2$D). Interestingly, all the steps in vitamin D metabolism are catalyzed by P_{450} enzymes (Allgrove, 2009).

If you look carefully, you will appreciate that vitamin D is a 9, 10-secosteroid (preporhormone), and because of this, it is treated as a hormone in the numbering of its carbon skeleton. Vitamin D exists in two distinct forms—vitamin D_2 and vitamin D_3. It is important to understand that vitamin D_3 is a **27**-carbon cholesterol derivative (the form manufactured by animals), whereas vitamin D_2 is a **28**-carbon molecule derived from the plant sterol ergosterol. Besides containing an extra methyl group, vitamin D_2 also differs from vitamin D_3 in that it contains a double bond between carbons 22 and 23.

The most important aspects of vitamin D chemistry center on its cistriene structure. This structure confers upon vitamin D a characteristic maximum ultraviolet (UV) absorption at 265 nm and a minimum at 228 nm. This unique cistriene structure makes vitamin D and related metabolites susceptible to oxidation, UV light-induced conformation changes, heat-induced conformation changes, and free radical attack. As a rule, the majority of these transformation products have lower biologic activity than does vitamin D. It is important to note that in humans, vitamins D_2 and D_3 are used interchangeably; as a result, unless otherwise noted, in this book the term vitamin D will refer to both compounds.

Metabolic activation of vitamin D is achieved through sequential hydroxylation reactions—first at the carbon 25 of the side chain and then the carbon 1 of the A ring. Metabolic inactivation of vitamin D takes place primarily through a series of oxidative reactions at carbons 23, 24, and 26 of the side chain of the molecule (see **Figure 1** for more detail). These metabolic activations and inactivations will be dealt with later in this section.

Photochemical Production of Vitamin D_3

Vitamin D_3 is produced in the skin from the provitamin D_3, 7-dehydrocholesterol (Esvelt et al., 1978; MacLaughlin & Holick, 1983). 7-dehydrocholesterol is distributed throughout the epidermis and dermis with highest concentrations in the stratum spinosum and stratum basale (Holick et al., 1980) Exposure of skin to sunlight, specifically to the UVB range of the spectrum (270-300 nm), results in the photolytic conversion of 7-dehydrocholesterol to previtamin D_3. Previtamin D_3 is transformed to vitamin D_3 by a thermally induced isomerization (**Figure 2**) (Esvelt et al., 1978). The production of vitamin D_3 is thought to be regulated by the amount of UV light reaching the 7-dehydrocholesterol, rather than by hormonal feedback (Matsuoka, Wortsman, & Hollis, 1988). It is interesting that vitamin D intoxication has never been reported because of excessive exposure to sunlight. Even in lifeguards, the concentration of serum 25-hydroxyvitamin D (25[OHJD) rarely exceeds 70 ng/mL (Haddad & Stamp, 1974), well within the safe range for this vitamin D metabolite.

For the skin to produce vitamin D, a threshold of 18-20 mJ/cm^2 of ultraviolet B light is required (Matsuoka et al., 1989). Sunscreen of SPF 8 or higher blocks vitamin D production (Matsuoka et al., 1987; Matsuoka, Wortsman, Hanifan & Holick, 1988; Matsuoka, Wortsman, & Hollis, 1990b; Holick, 1992; Holick, 1994). Cutaneous melanin content, the extent of which is dependent on race, limits the production of vitamin D (Matsuoka et al., 1991). In addition, the threshold of 18-20 mJ/cm^2 is not generally reached during the winter in northern United States above latitude 40°, regardless of pigmentation (Webb, Kline, & Holick, 1988). For example, in Boston (42° N latitude) in January, as Dr. Holick will attest (Holick, 1994), a Caucasian individual in a bathing suit outside on a sunny day will have no cutaneous production of vitamin D (Webb et al., 1988; Matsuoka et al., 1989). In comparison, that same individual in a bathing suit during the summer months can produce adequate vitamin D (~10,000-20,000 IU vitamin D) with 10-12 minutes of sun exposure (Matsuoka et al., 1989; Matsuoka, Wortsman, & Hollis, 1990a). An individual with darker pigmentation would need 60-72 minutes of exposure to synthesize the same amount of vitamin D (Clemens, Henderson, Adams, & Holick, 1982; Matsuoka, Wortsman, Haddad, & Hollis, 1990). This difference partly explains the racial disparities that we see with vitamin D status throughout the world: it takes more sunlight to achieve the same level in the blood because melanin acts as an excellent natural sunscreen (Matsuoka et al., 1991). This is not an issue if you live at the equator, but living at higher altitudes increases the risk of sunlight-derived vitamin D deficiency.

Control Processes Within the Body for Sun-Derived Vitamin D

The question of how the production of vitamin D_3 is limited in the face of excessive UV irradiation and a continuous supply of precursor, 7-dehydrocholesterol, is partially solved when taking into account the ability of the body to produce biologically inactive forms of vitamin D from the active precursors. On exposure to additional sunlight, previtamin D_3 is transformed not only into vitamin D_3, but also into lumesterol or tachysterol, which are both biologically inactive. This process is regulated and results in a reduction of the amount of previtamin D_3 that would be available for conversion to vitamin D_3. It is also known that excess sunlight can degrade vitamin D_3 into inert photoproducts, including suprasterols I and II (Webb, deCosta, & Holick, 1989). This mechanism further limits the amount of vitamin D_3 available after excessive exposure to sunlight. A number of other factors can limit or regulate the cutaneous production of vitamin D_3, including the use of sunscreens (Matsuoka et al., 1987), aging (MacLaughlin & Holick, 1985), increased melanin pigmentation (Holick, MacLaughlin, & Doppelt, 1981b), season of the year (Webb et al., 1988; Sherman, Hollis, & Tobin, 1990), and latitude (Webb et al., 1988). Each of these factors individually and in combination can influence the amount of vitamin D_3 released into the circulation and its further metabolism to more bioactive compounds.

Absorption of Vitamin D

In addition to its biosynthesis in the skin, vitamin D_3, along with vitamin D_2, can be obtained from the diet. Vitamin D is distributed very poorly in natural foodstuffs and is found primarily in fish oils, egg yolk, butter, and liver. Because of its low abundance, vitamin D is commonly fortified at low concentrations in food products, the most common product being milk. The amount of vitamin D normally added to milk products is 400 IU/quart—twice the current Adequate Intake (AI) for non-pregnant adults (200 IU/day) and equivalent to the current

AI for children and pregnant and lactating women (400 IU/day). The adequacy of this AI is in serious question (Hollis, 2005; Hollis, Wagner, Drezner, & Binkley, 2007). It should be noted that fortification of the milk supply with vitamin D tends to be a rather erratic practice, with variability in the amount actually present, with both ends of the spectrum represented—from very low to potentially toxic amounts of the vitamin in fortified milk (Tanner et al., 1988; Holick, Shao, Liu, & Chen, 1992; Jacobus et al., 1992). In fact, erratic fortification led to development of hypercalcemia as a consequence of vitamin D intoxication (Jacobus et al., 1992). Less evident would be cases of insufficient vitamin D intake by individuals ingesting milk products with low fortification. This could lead to vitamin D deficiency, osteomalacia, and rickets (Chapuy et al., 1992).

As with most fat-soluble compounds, vitamin D absorption takes place primarily in the upper portion of the small intestine where the pancreas and gallbladder contribute bile salts and digestive enzymes to process the fat component of foods. The aqueous environment of the intestinal lumen poses a major obstacle to the absorption of fat and fat-soluble vitamins. Formation of mixed micelles is accomplished by interaction of bile acids with lipids, including vitamin D. This step is a prerequisite for solubilization of vitamin D into an aqueous phase from which it can be absorbed by enterocytes (Wever, 1981). Vitamin D is absorbed by enterocytes by a non-saturable passive bile salt-dependent diffusion process (Hollander, Muralidhara, & Zimmerman, 1978). It is important to note, however, that although some of it is reabsorbed in the small intestine (Kumar, Nagubandi, & Londowski, 1980; Kumar, Nagubandi, Mattox & Londowski, 1980; Nagubandi, Kumar, Londowski, Corradino, & Tietz, 1980), the enterohepatic circulation of vitamin D is not considered to be an important mechanism for its conservation (Fraser, 1983). Additional processing occurs through formation of a variety of vitamin D's water metabolites, most notably calcitroic acid, which are excreted by the kidney into the urine (Esvelt & De Luca, 1981).

Experiments in healthy subjects show that, after ingestion of a single bolus of vitamin D_2, the circulating values of this compound begin to increase by 4 hours, are maximal at 8 hours, and return to near basal levels by 2 days (Haddad, Matsuoka, Hollis, Hu, & Wortsman, 1993). In contrast, patients with malabsorption syndromes, such as biliary atresia or cystic fibrosis, may be unable to absorb vitamin D (see the following section) (Heubi, Hollis, Specker, & Tsang, 1989; Heubi, Hollis, & Tsang, 1990). In addition to disease states, age itself is also known to have a negative effect on the absorption of lipophilic compounds (Barragry, France, et al., 1978). Thus, the elderly or those with certain hepatic or intestinal disease are susceptible to vitamin D deficiency. It should be noted, however, that malabsorption can be overcome to some degree by administration of a more hydrophilic form of vitamin D, such as $25(OH)D_3$ (Heubi et al., 1989), or by suspending vitamin D in a better solubilizing carrier that can aid its absorption (Argao, Heubi, Hollis, & Tsang, 1992).

Transport of Vitamin D

Once vitamin D enters the circulation from the skin or from the lymph via the thoracic duct, it accumulates in the liver within a few hours. Vitamin D and its metabolites are transported in the circulation bound principally to the vitamin D-binding protein (DBP). DBP is structurally related to albumin and α-fetoprotein, and not surprising given this relationship, is a member of the albumin and α-fetoprotein gene family (Cooke & David, 1985). The message for human DBP is made up of 1690 nucleotides and encodes a 458-amino acid secreted protein, and the gene for DBP contains 13 exons. The chromosome locus is 4q11-q13. Human plasma DBP is a 58,000-dalton, single-chain polypeptide that constitutes about 6 percent of the α-globulins in plasma (Guoth et al., 1990). Its concentration in serum is 4 to 8 µM, with a serum half-life of 2.5 to 3.0 days (Haddad, 1992).

Now that formalities about DBP are out of the way, we can focus on what it really does—it is the shuttle for vitamin D and its metabolites. DBP binds vitamin D and its metabolites with varying affinity that is based on the number and position of polar functional groups and/or methyl groups (Hollis, 1984). DBP has a high-affinity binding site for 25(OH)D (the dissociation constant Kd = 5×10^{-8}M), and preferentially binds 25(OH)D; $24,25(OH)_2D$; and $25,26(OH)_2D$, rather than $1,25(OH)_2D$ or its vitamin D parent compound (Hollis 1984). DBP binds vitamin D_2 metabolites with less affinity than those of vitamin D_3; however, clinically, they are viewed as equivalent in raising and maintaining vitamin D status as measured by circulating 25(OH)D (Holick et al., 2008). Circulating values for DBP are reduced in liver disease and are increased by pregnancy and estrogen, yet the serum concentration is not changed by vitamin D excess or deficiency (Barragry, Corless, et al., 1978). The high affinity of DBP for vitamin D metabolites coupled with the excessive binding capacity render "free" or unbound vitamin D and its metabolites to very low concentrations (Bikle et al., 1986). **This is important because only the "free" concentration of the vitamin is available to exert its biologic function. Those conditions that alter circulating concentrations of DBP (such as liver disease, pregnancy, increased estrogen states) also affect the "free" concentration of the vitamin.**

Mice without the gene for DBP [i.e., knockout mice of the *DBP* gene (DBP-/-)] are phenotypically normal, despite having undetectable serum DBP, and low serum 25(OH)D and $1,25(OH)_2D$. DBP negative mice are at risk for developing rickets when vitamin D is restricted and are resistant to excess vitamin D (Safadi et al., 1999). Radiolabeled $25(OH)D_3$ is cleared rapidly from the circulation of these DBP-/- mice. We can decipher the role of DBP from such studies: DBP functions to sequester vitamin D and its metabolites into the circulation, to prolong their half-lives, and perhaps, most relevant to modern society, to provide a storehouse of vitamin D during episodes of vitamin D deficiency.

DBP is important with respect to the transport and tissue delivery of vitamin D after cutaneous or dietary supplementation. Distinct differences are recognized with respect to transport of vitamin D derived from cutaneous synthesis versus vitamin D derived from the diet: when compared to the effect of oral vitamin D administration, it appears that a more efficient and sustained supply of vitamin D is associated with UV irradiation of the skin (Haddad et al., 1993). In contrast to cutaneous synthesis of vitamin D, oral vitamin D leads to a more rapid, but decreased, sustained availability of vitamin D. Haddad et al. demonstrated that vitamin D generated by cutaneous production is almost entirely associated with DBP on entrance into the circulation, whereas orally administered vitamin D_2 is equally distributed between DBP and lipoproteins on entry into the circulation. This observation is significant in that cutaneous production of vitamin D_3 would result in a gradual and more sustained plasma availability of vitamin D and 25(OH)D. Rapid hepatic delivery of vitamin D can result in its waste, with the appearance of inactive forms, including its water-soluble conjugates (Litwiller et al., 1982).

Why is this important? From a physiologic standpoint, through evolution, vitamin D was intended to be released from the skin associated with high-affinity DBP for subsequent delivery to the liver (Hollis, 2005). Oral delivery of the vitamin through naturally occurring foods was a minimal contributor, except for certain areas of the world, such as the Arctic Circle, where individuals subsisted on marine animals, such as whale, seal, and polar bear. For the vast majority of humans during the last several thousand years, oral vitamin D was likely a non-physiologic phenomenon, given its association in the circulation with low-affinity carriers (Haddad et al., 1993) that are unregulated and could result in serious toxicity (Jacobus et al., 1992).

Comparison of Sun-Derived Versus Oral Vitamin D Supplementation

The relative inefficiency of dietary contribution to overall vitamin D status is shown by the following: If sunlight exposure is halved, the vitamin D intake must be tripled to compensate and maintain the same level of circulating 25(OH)D within the body (Allgrove, 2009). Since sunscreen, clothing, and lifestyles can significantly decrease sunlight exposure; despite its limitations, dietary supplementation of vitamin D becomes a viable and, perhaps exclusive, option for a great majority of people in the 21st century.

A study by Hollis et al. (2007) compared vitamin D derived from the sun and from oral supplementation. Individuals who reported daily sun exposure of at least >15 hours peak sun exposure/week were compared with our pilot study of fully lactating women randomized to either 400 or 6400 IU vitamin D/day (Wagner et al., 2006). In this study, the following differences were noted:

(1) Despite reporting more than 15 hours of sunlight exposure per week, there was much variability in the 25(OH)D levels in the sun-exposure group, as some had limited surface area exposure—with only hands and head exposed (e.g., in those who surfed with wetsuits). Thus, one can be vitamin D deficient with significant sun exposure if the skin area exposed is limited.

(2) The relationship between circulating vitamin D and 25(OH)D is not linear, but is saturable and controlled.

(3) Optimal nutritional vitamin D status may occur when equamolar levels of circulating vitamin D_3 and 25(OH)D_3 occur (>40 ng/mL); at this point, the V_{max} of the enzyme appears to be achieved.[8]

(4) Whether one receives their vitamin D_3 orally or through UV exposure, the vitamin D-25-hydroxylase handles it in an equivalent fashion (Hollis et al., 2007).

The third point above—that optimal vitamin D status may occur when equal concentrations of circulating vitamin D and 25(OH)D occur above 40 ng/mL (100 nmol/L)—is interesting, as this finding sheds light on the enzyme kinetics of vitamin D 25-hydroxylase. As humans live today, this enzyme operates below its V_{max} because of the chronic deficiency of substrate vitamin D. Not a single other steroidal hormone system in the body is limited in this fashion since their starting point is cholesterol (Hollis et al., 2007). When humans are sun (or dietary) replete, the vitamin D system will function in a fashion as do our other steroid synthetic pathways, i.e., not limited by substrate availability.

---

[8] Because enzymes are biological catalysts, they speed up chemical reactions. The speed of any particular reaction or rate being catalyzed by a particular enzyme can only reach a certain maximum value, and this rate is known as V_{max}. The precise definition of V_{max} is the maximum initial velocity of the enzyme catalyzed reaction under the given conditions. It is the limiting value that the initial rate of reaction V_o approaches as the substrate concentration approaches infinity. V_o has to be used because the rate of some reactions decreases with time due to things like feedback inhibition. Lastly, V_{max} is measured in units of quantity of substrate transformed per unit time for a given concentration of enzyme.

7. METABOLISM OF VITAMIN D

By Bruce W. Hollis, Ph.D. and Carol L. Wagner, M.D.

For those of you who disdain anything with a chemical symbol or reaction, this may not be the section for you. Yet, you might be surprised. Empower yourself with the knowledge that not only does structure beget function, but as that structure changes, the function and role of that protein, that hormone—in this case, vitamin D—within the body changes. For those who want to understand the metabolism of vitamin D and what is happening within the body, this section is for you.

Factors Influencing Vitamin D Status

Before one can undertake any discussion about vitamin D metabolism, one must consider those factors that impact the vitamin D that circulates within the body, because without this substrate, there is no metabolic processing of vitamin D. Perhaps the single most important factor in determining your vitamin D status is sunlight exposure. It accounts for more than 80% of your body's total vitamin D (Matsuoka et al., 1989). A close second to sunlight are those collective factors that determine your sunlight exposure—degree of skin pigmentation, clothing, use of sunscreen, and actual time spent outdoors or under an ultraviolet B light source with skin exposure.

The darker the pigmentation, the more ultraviolet light is needed to activate the photochemical processes in the skin. An increase in skin melanin pigmentation or the topical application of a sunscreen will absorb solar ultraviolet B photons, which significantly reduces the production of vitamin D_3 in the skin (Clemens et al., 1982; Matsuoka et al., 1987; Matsuoka, Wortsman, Hanifan, et al., 1988). Melanin absorbs ultraviolet light from ~270-315 nm, but the melanin and its melanopores that determine skin color are situated in the skin above the keratinocytes that actually synthesize vitamin D_3. The more melanin above (acting as a filter in the way that sunscreen acts) means there is a greater absorption of ultraviolet light hitting the surface of the skin that does not reach the keratinocytes below. Thus, darker pigmented individuals require a greater degree of sunlight exposure to achieve the same effect as lighter pigmented individuals with less melanin. Once the vitamin D_3 is synthesized, there are no differences in metabolism of vitamin D or processing within the body per se (Lo, Paris, & Holick, 1986; Matsuoka, Wortsman, Haddad, et al., 1990).

Beyond an individual's given skin pigmentation, there are universal factors that determine how much vitamin D will ultimately be synthesized by the skin. Body surface area exposed is an important component. For example, exposure of your trunk, which has the largest surface area, will yield more vitamin D after a comparable period of time than your face and hands, which have comparatively little surface area. One of the folk doctrines that often is espoused by many in medicine is that if you put your face and hands out the window for 15 minutes a few times per week, this sunlight exposure will generate enough vitamin D to keep you in the sufficient range (Matsuoka, Wortsman, Hanifan, et al., 1988; Matsuoka et al., 1989; Matsuoka, Wortsman, Haddad, et al., 1990; Matsuoka, Wortsman, et al., 1990a; Matsuoka, Wortsman, et al., 1990b; Matsuoka et al., 1991; Matsuoka et al., 1992). Unless you live at the equator, this is fallacious thinking. Thus, sunlight exposure's effect on the body's synthesis of vitamin D depends on the surface area of the body that is exposed (Matsuoka et al., 1989).

A corollary of body surface area is body mass index (BMI). Individuals with a higher BMI (>30) tend to have lower circulating 25(OH)D because the adipose tissue acts as a reservoir for vitamin D (Borissova, Tankova, Kirilov, Dakovska, & Kovacheva, 2003; Liu et al., 2005; Egan et al., 2008; Jacobs et al., 2008). In two recent studies involving obese patients, BMI and vitamin D status were inversely related. In a study by McGill et al., serum vitamin D_3 was inversely related to weight, BMI, and markers of Type 2 insulin-dependent diabetes (IDM) (large waist, raised HbA1c), but not to adipose mass or metabolic syndrome per se (McGill, Stewart, Lithander, Strik, & Poppitt, 2008). Lagunova et al., in their study of 2,126 patients registered in a Metabolic and Medical Lifestyle Management Clinic in Oslo, Norway, measured circulating 25(OH)D and 1,25(OH)$_2$D levels. Seasonal variation and prevalence of vitamin D deficiency were assessed in different body mass index (BMI), sex, and age categories (Lagunova, Porojnicu, Lindberg,

Hexeberg, & Moan, 2009). They found that for both men and women and across the lifespan (<50 years and ≥50 years), there was a significant decrease of serum 25(OH)D$_3$ and serum 1,25(OH)$_2$D$_3$ levels with increasing BMI. The seasonal variation of serum 25(OH)D$_3$ was highest in young (<50 years), non-obese men. The prevalence of vitamin D deficiency was highest in individuals with BMI ≥40, being as high as 32% among women and 46% among men. In this large cohort study of individuals living in Norway, the risk of vitamin D deficiency occurred in 1 in 3 women and 1 in 2 men with BMI ≥40 (Lagunova et al., 2009). While the risk of vitamin D deficiency is higher at this latitude due to diminished sunlight and a reduced capacity to synthesize vitamin D for more than 6 months of the year, higher BMI and lower vitamin D levels are found at any latitude (Egan et al., 2008; Jacobs et al., 2008).

Seasonality is another important issue: during winter months for many parts of the world, the angle of the sun is altered such that the UVB that reaches the skin is below the necessary range for vitamin D synthesis (Holick, 1995a). As the seasons change from summer to late fall, the angle of the sun changes and time of day of exposure also matters. Latitude, time of day, and season of the year have a dramatic influence on the cutaneous production of vitamin D$_3$. Above and below latitudes of approximately 40° N and 40° S, respectively, vitamin D$_3$ synthesis in the skin is absent during most of the three to four winter months (Webb et al., 1988; Ladizesky et al., 1995), and those more northern and southern latitudes beyond extend this period of absent vitamin D synthesis for up to 6 months (Oliveri, Ladizesky, Mautalen, Alonso, & Martinez, 1993; Holick, 1994). In this way, both latitude and season play significant roles. One does not need to worry about seasonality per se in areas of the world nearest the equator—of course, assuming that an individual's skin is exposed to sunlight.

The amount of clothing while in the sun is another factor that will determine your vitamin D status (Matsuoka et al., 1992). If your skin is covered for cultural or religious reasons, then you are at greatest risk of developing vitamin D deficiency, and so, too, during pregnancy, your fetus is at risk of developing vitamin D deficiency, and once born, if you breastfeed, your infant is at greatest risk of developing vitamin D deficiency. Sunscreen acts like clothing and a Sun Protective Factor (SPF) of 8 or greater will act to block the ultraviolet light from reaching the keratinocytes of the epidermis necessary for the photochemical reaction to make vitamin D (Matsuoka, Wortsman, et al., 1990b; Matsuoka et al., 1992).

Processing of Vitamin D Within the Body

As discussed in **Section 6**, once vitamin D enters the circulation (**Figure 2**), either through epidermal transfer or intestinal absorption, it associates with vitamin D-binding protein (DBP) (Hollis, 1984) and is transported to the liver. It is in the liver that the initial step in the metabolic activation of vitamin D takes place. Vitamin D—either vitamin D_2 or D_3— comes in contact with the 25-hydroxylase enzyme that initiates hydroxylation at carbon 25. While this reaction can take place in various cells in the body, this oxidation process is primarily a hepatic function that results in the production of 25(OH)D, the most abundant circulating form of vitamin D (Bhattacharyya & Deluca, 1974; Haddad & Stamp 1974). Bhattacharyya and DeLuca (1974) first identified liver microsomes as a site of 25-hydroxylation of vitamin D_3. Subsequently, Bjorkhem and Holmberg (1978) demonstrated that the 25-hydroxylation of vitamin D_3 occurred in both the microsomal and mitochondrial fractions of the liver. The enzyme vitamin D-25-hydroxylase is a cytochrome P_{450} mixed-function oxidase that is nicotinamide adenine dinucleotide phosphate (NADP)-dependent (Madhok & DeLuca, 1979). Subsequent studies have focused on the enzyme kinetics of the 25-hydroxylases contained in both the microsomes and mitochondria (Bjorkhem & Holmberg, 1978; Delvin, Arabian, & Glorieux, 1978; Madhok, Schnoes, & DeLuca, 1978; Madhok & DeLuca, 1979).

There are four known enzymes that have an influence on 25(OH)D hydroxylase activity, which can be distinguished by their different affinities and capacities to induce 25(OH)D hydroxylase, as well as their intracellular localization (Allgrove, 2009). The first, a low-affinity, high capacity enzyme called CYP27A1 is found in the mitochondria involved in the formation of bile acids from cholesterol. This enzyme appears to have limited physiologic importance with respect to vitamin D metabolism, and leads one to question whether this 25-hydroxylase is a true vitamin D-metabolizing enzyme or a cholesterol-metabolizing enzyme that happens to recognize the cholesterol side-chain of vitamin D_3.[9] The second enzyme, CYP2R1, is a high-affinity, low-capacity enzyme for both vitamin D_2 and vitamin D_3 that is located in hepatic microsomes, and which appears to have greater physiological significance than the other three enzymes (Cheng, Motola, Mangelsdorf, & Russell, 2003; Allgrove, 2009). The third and fourth enzymes— CYP3A4 and CYP2J2— have only partial effect as 25-hydroxylases, with their main function appearing to be drug metabolism (Allgrove, 2009).

While the tissue distribution of vitamin D-25-hydroxylase appears to be diverse (Tucker, Gagnon, & Haussler, 1973), it is generally agreed that the liver is the major site of this enzyme (Olson, Knutson, Bhattacharyya & DeLuca, 1976). Very little is known about the metabolic control of this enzyme. Regulation of 25(OH)D production is difficult to demonstrate because excessive administration of vitamin D results in marked increases in serum 25(OH)D and vitamin D toxicity. Whereas 1,25(OH)$_2$D is thought to inhibit the hepatic production of 25(OH)D (Bell, Shaw, & Turner, 1984), the ability of 1,25(OH)$_2$D to reduce circulating 25(OH)D is mediated by increasing the metabolic clearance and metabolism of 25(OH)D through activation of 25(OH)D-24-hydroxylase.

Anti-convulsant drugs tend to reduce circulating 25(OH)D by increasing the catabolism or breakdown of 25(OH)D (Hahn & Halstead, 1979). As mentioned earlier, hepatic disease, such as biliary atresia, and cystic fibrosis also lead to reduced serum 25(OH)D as a consequence of impaired intestinal absorption of fats, which includes vitamin D (Heubi et al., 1989). Because anti-convulsants affect liver function, there are changes in vitamin D metabolism, such that even if that individual had adequate sunlight exposure, the hepatic conversion of vitamin D_3 to 25(OH)D would be hindered. In comparison, in patients with fat malabsorption, but with adequate liver function, endogenous synthesis of vitamin D by the skin

---

[9] Evidence of this enzyme's limited physiologic importance: (1) The dissociation constant of the enzyme (Km) is very high (in the range of 1 M). (2) The enzyme has never been shown to 25-hydroxylate vitamin D_2, a function the true vitamin D-25 hydroxylase would have to perform. (This premise is supported by an *in vitro* experiment where mitochondrial 25-hydroxylase was isolated, purified, sequenced, transfected, and expressed in COS-1 cells, where it catalyzed hydroxylation of vitamin D_3, but not D_2 (Guo et al., 1993). (3) Patients with deficiency of 25-hydroxylase (CYP27) develop something called cerebrotendinous xanthomatosis and not rickets (Cali et al., 1991). (4) Mice with knock-out CYP27 have one-fold increases in serum 25(OH)D, and not deficiencies of circulating 25(OH)D (Rosen,et al., 1998).

through sunlight exposure would still be possible (Stamp, Haddad, & Twigg, 1977; Esvelt et al., 1978; Holick, MacLaughlin, & Doppelt, 1981a; Aris et al., 2005). While there are dangers associated with UV exposure (1999), in those individuals with fat malabsorption, sunlight or UV exposure becomes their primary source of vitamin D (Hahn & Halstead, 1979; Lark et al., 2001; Aris et al., 2005).

After its formation in the liver, 25(OH)D appears in the circulation bound primarily to DBP. The half-life of 25(OH)D in the circulation is about 2 to 3 weeks in normal individuals (Smith & Goodman, 1971). **Because of its relatively long half-life compared to that of vitamin D and other polar metabolites, circulating 25(OH)D is *the* indicator of nutritional vitamin D status** (Haddad & Stamp, 1974; Hollis et al., 2007) **and can be measured by a variety of analytical methods** (Haddad & Chyu, 1971; Eisman, Shepard, & Deluca, 1977; Hollis et al., 1993). While a reduction in the concentration of serum 25(OH)D occasionally occurs in the nephritic syndrome, sarcoidosis, tuberculosis, hyperphosphatemic tumoral calcinosis, primary hyperparathyroidism, and vitamin D-dependent rickets type II as a consequence of increased serum $1,25(OH)_2D$, it is more frequently normal in these disorders.

The Active Hormone $1,25(OH)_2D$

In order to have biologic activity at physiologic concentrations, 25(OH)D must be hydroxylated on the 1-carbon position to form $1,25(OH)_2D$ (Holick, Schnoes, DeLuca, Suda, et al., 1971; Omdahl, Holick, Suda, Tanaka, & DeLuca, 1971); this is true in the kidney and in the extrarenal tissues throughout the body. It is also true that the primary site of regulation of vitamin D metabolism is the kidney. In the kidney, $1,25(OH)_2D$ and $24,25(OH)_2D$ are produced by cytochrome P_{450} mixed-function oxidases in the mitochondria of the proximal tubules (Ghazarian, Jefcoate, Knutson, Orme-Johnson & Deluca, 1974). The kidney, however, is not limited to the production of these two compounds because many other metabolites are produced in this organ. The physiologic relevance, if any, of these many compounds remains unknown. Therefore, metabolism of only the two predominant metabolites, $1,25(OH)_2D$ and $24,25(OH)_2D$, will be discussed below.

As with the liver's vitamin D-25-hydroxylase, both the 25(OH)D-1α- and 25(OH)D-24-hydroxylases require molecular oxygen and a source of reducing equivalents to hydroxylate positions 1α or 24R of 25(OH)D (Ghazarian et al., 1974). The substrate specificity of the 1α-hydroxylase is highest for 25(OH)D, but other metabolites, such as $24,25(OH)_2D$ and $25,26(OH)_2D$, can be 1α-hydroxylated to yield compounds with significant biologic activity (Boris, Hurley, & Trmal, 1977). Conversely, the 1α-hydroxylase cannot 1α-hydroxylate the parent compound vitamin D.

Within the kidney, the 1α-hydroxylase was shown to be located in two distinct sites: the proximal convoluted tubules and the pars recta (Akiba et al., 1980). The 1α-hydroxylase of the proximal convoluted tubule is stimulated by parathyroid hormone, whereas the 1α-hydroxylase in the pars recta is increased by calcitonin, leading to two discrete loci of control of the conversion to the active hormone (Kawashima, Torikai, & Kurokawa, 1981a; Kawashima, Torikai, & Kurokawa, 1981b; Kawashima & Kurokawa, 1982).

It is $1,25(OH)_2D$ that is the biologically active form of vitamin D and which appears to be responsible for most, if not all, of its biologic functions (Holick, Schnoes, DeLuca, Suda, & Cousins, 1971; Holick, Schnoes, & DeLuca, 1971; Omdahl et al., 1971; Tanaka, DeLuca, Omdahl, & Holick, 1971; Garabedian, Pavlovitch, Fellot, & Balsan, 1974; Garabedian, Tanaka, Holick & Deluca, 1974; Fraser, 1980; DeLuca, 1988; Reichel, Koeffler, & Norman, 1989; Reichel & Norman, 1989). It has been known for some time that the production of $1,25(OH)_2D$ in the kidney is tightly regulated, principally through the action of PTH in response to serum calcium and phosphorus levels (Portale, Booth, Halloran, & Morris, 1984; Reichel et al., 1989; Reichel & Norman, 1989). Because of the tight regulation of the production of $1,25(OH)_2D$ and its relatively short serum half-life of 4-6 hours (Kumar, Nagubandi, Mattox, et al., 1980), it has not proven to be a valuable marker for vitamin D deficiency, adequacy, or excess.

When dietary calcium intake is inadequate to satisfy the body's calcium requirement, $1,25(OH)_2D$, along with parathyroid hormone (PTH), mobilizes monocytic stem cells in the bone marrow to become mature osteoclasts (Merke, Klaus, Hugel, Waldherr, & Ritz, 1986; Holick, 1995). The osteoclasts, in turn, are stimulated by a variety of cytokines and other factors to increase the mobilization of calcium stores from the bone. In this manner, vitamin D facilitates the homeostasis of blood calcium and phosphorus at supersaturating concentrations that are deposited in the bone as calcium hydroxyapatite. *This relationship explains the findings of osteopenia or bone demineralization during states of vitamin D deficiency.*

Renal Regulation of Vitamin D Metabolism

In contrast to the hepatic vitamin D-25-hydroxylase enzymes, the activity of the renal 25(OH)-1α-hydroxylase is strictly regulated by calcium and phosphorus (Deluca, 1981), and to a lesser degree by other circulating factors. This strict regulation is necessitated by the extremely high biopotency of $1,25(OH)_2D$. $1,25(OH)_2D$, which acts primarily through its nuclear receptor (VDR) in target tissues, is at least 1,000-fold more bioactive as compared to its precursor, 25(OH) D. Regulation of the renal 25(OH)D-1α-hydroxylase by calcium is thought to be mediated by parathyroid hormone (PTH) through a cyclic adenosine monophosphate-dependent mechanism, although some studies suggest a direct role for calcium in the regulation of enzyme activity (Garabedian, Holick, Deluca & Boyle, 1972; Favus & Long, 1986) mediated through the calcium receptor (Brown & Hebert, 1997). Other *in vitro* studies using cultured chick kidney cells also suggest a possible role for protein kinase C in down-regulation of 25(OH) D-1α -hydroxylase activity (Favus & Long, 1986).

In view of the possible role of protein kinases in regulation of the 25(OH)D-1α-hydroxylase, some studies have attempted to determine whether phosphorylation of the cytochrome P_{450} itself or one of the other components plays a role in the regulation of the enzyme. Based on studies with the chicken enzyme, it would appear that phosphorylation of the cytochrome P_{450} component has no effect on enzyme activity, whereas phosphorylation of the ferredoxin component inhibits 25(OH)D-1α-hydroxylase activity in a reconstituted system (Garabedian et al., 1972; Nemani et al., 1989). Based on these and other studies, a model for regulation of the renal α-hydroxylase involving phosphorylation and dephosphorylation of the ferredoxin component was proposed (Ghazarian, 1990; Mandel, Moorthy, & Ghazarian, 1990).

Regulation of the renal 1α-hydroxylase by phosphate apparently is not mediated by parathyroid hormone, but is dependent upon growth hormone and may be mediated by insulin-like growth factor (IGF-1) (Gray, Garthwaite, & Phillips, 1983). However, because concentrations of IGF-1 in serum and renal tissue do not change during phosphate deprivation, the function of this growth factor in mediating the low phosphate stimulation of the 25(OH)D-1α-hydroxylase may be permissive (Gray et al., 1983; Gray, 1987). It was suggested that IGF-1 enhances renal tubular phosphate flux, which may, in turn, influence the activity of the 25(OH)D-1α-hydroxylase (Caverzasio, Montessuit, & Bonjour, 1990). Unlike the effects of parathyroid hormone, which can be studied *in vitro*, a direct effect of phosphate on the renal 25(OH)D-1α -hydroxylase *in vitro* has been difficult to demonstrate reproducibly, thus making it difficult to study the mechanism of this effect.

Another potent regulator of renal 25(OH)D-1α-hydroxylase activity is $1,25(OH)_2D$ itself (Hollis, Roos, & Lambert, 1980). It was demonstrated several years ago that administration of exogenous $1,25(OH)_2D$, would stimulate the catabolic cascade of renal enzymes involved in the metabolism of 25(OH)D (Hollis, Roos, et al., 1980). Additional studies showed $1,25(OH)_2D$ to be an effective down-regulator of renal 25(OH)D-1α-hydroxylase activity (Fox, Kollenkirchen, & Walters, 1991). This down-regulation was shown to occur through both non-genomic mechanisms (Dick, Retallack, & Prince, 1990) and proposed genomic alterations of the enzyme (Fox et al. 1991), which indirectly supports the premise that vitamin D and its metabolites exert epigenetic controls (Kussmann & Affolter, 2009). Other factors are also thought to affect renal 25(OH)D-1α-hydroxylase activity, although their mode of control is far from complete.

Extrarenal Metabolism of 25(OH)D

Although we know most about liver and renal effects, cell surface receptors that recognize both $1,25(OH)_2D$ and 25(OH)D abound throughout the body, including the brain, heart, pancreas, mononuclear cells, activated lymphocytes, and skin (Stumpf, Sar, Reid, Tanaka, & DeLuca, 1979; Lambert et al., 1982; Stumpf, Clark, Sar, & DeLuca, 1984; Turner, Avioli, & Bell, 1984; Stumpf, Clark, O'Brien, & Reid, 1988). The exact physiologic function of $1,25(OH)_2D$

in these diverse organs and cells is not fully elucidated, but it appears to act as a potent antiproliferative and prodifferentiation hormone (Abe et al., 1981; Colston, Colston, & Feldman, 1981; Eisman et al., 1981; Sher, Eisman, Moseley, & Martin, 1981). Until recently, it was thought that there was little evidence that vitamin D deficiency leads to major disorders in these organ and cellular systems. With enhanced molecular techniques, the role of vitamin D in extrarenal tissues has been demonstrated.

This aspect of vitamin D metabolism continues to emerge as important as its renal metabolism. The technical ability to be able to clone and characterize human 25(OH) D-1α-hydroxylase (CYP-1α) led to a number of studies to assess potential extrarenal conversion of vitamin D (Letterio & Roberts 1997). A number of studies in recent years demonstrated that the kidney is not the only tissue that produces 1,25(OH)$_2$D. Placenta (Gray, Lester, & Lorenc, 1979), bone cells (Howard, Turner, Sherrard, & Baylink, 1981), activated alveolar macrophages (Adams & Gacad, 1985), keratinocytes (Bikle et al., 1986; Veenstra et al., 1998; Eyles, Smith, Kinobeb, Hewison, & McGrath, 2005), prostate (Mikhak et al., 2007) and liver tissue (Hollis, 1990), to name a few, express 1α-hydroxylase activity *in vitro* (Turner et al., 1984; Zehnder et al., 2001). The finding of excessive, unregulated production of 1,25(OH)$_2$D by activated macrophages and lymphoma cells is responsible for the hypercalciuria associated with chronic granulomatous disorders and the hypercalcemia seen with lymphoma (Adams, 1989; Adams et al., 1989; Davies, Hayes, Yin, Berry, & Mawer, 1994). Whether these extrarenal tissues contribute 1,25(OH)$_2$D in an endocrine fashion is not established. What is known, however, is that anephric individuals have low, but clearly detectable serum concentrations of 1,25(OH)$_2$D and the values correlate with serum 25(OH)D (Lambert et al., 1982).

It is more likely that 1,25(OH)$_2$D produced by these tissues performs an autocrine, paracrine, or intracrine role in the tissues producing it, depending on the function of that tissue. In normal subjects, the major metabolite of 25(OH)D is 24,25(OH)$_2$D (Hollis & Pittard, 1984). As with 1,25(OH)$_2$D (Fraser & Kodicek, 1970), the kidney is the major site of production of 24,25(OH)$_2$D (Garabedian, Pavlovitch, et al., 1974), but its synthesis is known to occur in nearly all target tissues for 1,25(OH)$_2$D. The renal 25(OH)D-24-hydroxylase (*CYP24*) is similar to the

1α-hydroxylase in that it is located in the inner membrane of the mitochondria and is a cytochrome P_{450} monoxygenase. *CYP24* was isolated, sequenced, transfected, and expressed in COS cells (Ohyama, Noshiro, & Okuda, 1991). The coding region for the enzyme was shown to reside on human chromosome 20q 13.1 (Labuda, Lemieux, Tihy, Prinster, & Glorieux, 1993). The amino acid sequence of the 25(OH)D-24-hydroxylase demonstrates only a 30 percent homology with any of the previously sequenced cytochrome P_{450}'s (Ohyama et al., 1991), and is now known to be distinct from the renal 25(OH)-1α-hydroxylase (Akeno, Saikatsu, & Horiuchi, 1993; Arabian, Grover, Barre, & Delvin, 1993).

The actual function of the 25(OH)D-24-hydroxylase is controversial in that the biologic function of 24,25(OH),D is still unclear. Several reports attributed specific biologic actions to this metabolite, including stimulation of cellular membrane inositol 1,4,5-triphosphate (Grosse, Bourdeau, & Lieberherr, 1993); increase in bone volume (Nakamura, Suzuki, Hirai, Kurokawa, & Orimo, 1992); stimulation of calcification of cartilage matrix (Hinek & Poole, 1988), chondrocyte membrane alkaline phosphatase and phospholipase-A_2 (Schwartz, Bonewald, Caulfield, Brooks, & Boyan, 1993), and cytosolic-free calcium in osteoblasts (Lieberherr, 1987); and proliferation and differentiation of costal chondrocytes (Takigawa, Enomoto, Shirai, Nishii, & Suzuki, 1988). On the other hand, 24-hydroxylation of vitamin D metabolites was shown to be a first step in their degradation and excretion (Onisko, Esvelt, Schnoes, & DeLuca, 1980). Indeed, mice with knock-out of the *CYF24* gene develop hypercalcemia as a consequence of increased circulating 1,25(OH)$_2$D (St-Arnaud et al., 2000). It is clear that *CYP24* is the rate-limiting step in the degradation of biologically active metabolites of vitamin D.

Vitamin D Receptor (VDR)

The classic model for the action of steroid hormones proposes that the binding of the ligand to the receptor induces an allosteric change that allows the receptor hormone complex to bind to its DNA response element in the promoter region of a target gene. The DNA sequence analysis of vitamin D receptor (VDR) clones from chick (McDonnell, Mangelsdorf, Pike, Haussler, & O'Malley, 1987), human (Baker et al., 1988), and rat tissue (Evans, 1988) revealed extensive regions of very high homology that were considered to represent domains important in receptor function and several regions of lower homology. The similarity between the receptors indicates that the VDR is highly conserved across species and is an ancient and conserved receptor. The VDR is a polypeptide consisting of 424 amino acids with an N-terminal domain, amino acids 1 to 89 that bind DNA, a C-terminal domain, amino acids 182 to 427 that bind $1,25(OH)_2D$, and an intervening hinge, amino acids 89 to 182.

It is interesting that the conserved domains of VDR exhibit high sequence homology to glucocorticoid, progesterone, and estrogen receptors. This conservation indicates that these gene products belong to a superfamily of proteins whose functions are to mediate the genomic actions of their respective ligands (Evans, 1988). This aspect of the VDR helps explain its mode of action and its far-reaching effects on various systems throughout the body.

8. In Search Of The Holy Grail—What Does Vitamin D Really Do?

By Carol L. Wagner, M.D., Sarah N. Taylor, M.D., and Bruce W. Hollis, Ph.D.

Depending on the forum, the answer to the question posed by the title of this section is an elusive one. Some might say that vitamin D's chief importance is in calcium metabolism and bone metabolism; others might say that it is in immune function and preventing inflammation. The answer is both, with perhaps some overlap. In this section, we will focus on the first role of vitamin D—how it brings about an elevation of plasma calcium and phosphorus—and then we will discuss some of the latest findings about vitamin D's mediation of immune function during health and disease. As we delve into the functions of vitamin D, it is important to remind ourselves that almost 100 years ago Mellanby—during his experiments with rachitic dogs and in his observations of children—made the link between vitamin D and immune function. Yet, despite his careful observations, this aspect of his work went largely unnoticed. We should take heed of this tendency of ours—whether in science or in life—to gloss over those aspects of data or clinical presentations that do not fit our working paradigm—those facts unnoticed will remain until we learn from them, but as is the case with vitamin D, not without the dire consequences of such neglect and oversight.

Vitamin D, Calcium, and Phosphorus: Their Interrelation

According to Dr. Hector DeLuca, in his paper presented at the 71st Annual Meeting of the Federation of American Societies for Experimental Biology (FASEB), vitamin D brings about the elevation of calcium and phosphorus by way of three basic mechanisms (DeLuca, 1988):

(1) As the only known substance to stimulate enterocytes of the small intestine to transport calcium from the lumen to the plasma

compartment, vitamin D effects and directs the absorption of both calcium and phosphorus. Unlike in bone and in the kidney's distal proximal tubules where vitamin D acts with parathyroid hormone (PTH), in the intestine, vitamin D acts alone.

(2) Given the unreliability of diet to provide calcium, there must be a reservoir in the body of calcium. In addition to its role of providing support for vital organs and the morphotype of humans, the skeleton is a "sink hole" for calcium. To deposit or mobilize calcium in the skeleton, two hormones—vitamin D and PTH work in concert.

(3) Within the kidney, the distal renal tubules act to reabsorb calcium, an effect directed by both PTH and vitamin D that again must work in concert.

The circulating calcium concentration is sensed initially by the calcium-sensing receptor (CaSR), which in turn, results in a cascade of events that includes secretion of PTH—when circulating calcium concentration falls, it increases. PTH acts via a second messenger system on the target organs—principally bone and kidney. Abnormalities in any part of this system can cause a derangement in calcium, from hypocalcemia when there is vitamin D deficiency to hypercalcemia when there is hypervitaminosis D (Allgrove, 2009; Davies, 2009). The main systemic regulators of calcium homeostasis include PTH, $1,25(OH)_2D$ and, to a lesser extent, calcitonin (Allgrove, 2009; Davies, 2009). Under normal conditions, PTH stimulates the release of calcium from bone. It acts to promote reabsorption of calcium in the kidney's loop of Henle, and by stimulating renal 1α-hydroxylase activity, catalyzes the conversion of $25(OH)D$ to $1,25(OH)_2D$ (Allgrove, 2009; Davies, 2009).

Vitamin D and Its Role in both Innate and Adaptive Immunity

Mellanby noted poor health and immune dysfunction in the form of respiratory and skin infections and poor growth in the rachitic children of his day that was recapitulated in the rachitic dogs of his laboratory (Mellanby & Cantag, 1919; Mellanby, 1921). A few astute physicians had observed that children with rickets appeared ill, had less energy, and were more susceptible to respiratory illnesses (Weick, 1967; Rehman, 1994), but it was not until recently that the connection of vitamin D with immune function was refined down to the molecular level. Rook and colleagues first noted that $1,25(OH)_2D$ had noncalciotropic properties. Both $1,25(OH)_2D$ and $25(OH)D$ have the ability to induce the expression of cathelicidin in monocyte/macrophage and epidermal lineage in cells that simultaneously have CYP27B1—the $25(OH)D$ hydroxylase that itself requires cell-specific stimulation of Toll-like receptors (TLR2) (Bikle, Adams, & Christakos, 2008).[10] $1,25(OH)_2D$ not only has the ability to act intracellularly in macrophages and monocytes, but T and B lymphocytes as well. The presence of vitamin D receptor (VDR) in activated (but not resting) human T and B lymphocytes was the first observation made that implicated these cells as targets of $1,25(OH)_2D$ acting in a noncalciotropic (non-calcium metabolism) manner. Whereas $1,25(OH)_2D$ appears to activate the bacteriocidal process within macrophages and monocytes, it has the reverse effect in lymphocytes and appears to act in an anti-inflammatory manner.

The synthesis of two decades of work came together through the use of DNA array to characterize changes in gene expression after activation of a human macrophage TLR2/1 dimer by one of the pathogen-associated membrane proteins (PAMPs) for *M.* tuberculosis. It was known that cathelicidin (LL-37), an endogenous antimicrobial peptide generated by the innate immune system in response to microbial invasion, is activated through Toll 2 surface receptor activation on monocytes and macrophages (Liu et al., 2006; Liu, Stenger, Tang, & Modlin, 2007; Zheng et al., 2007). The vitamin D receptor (VDRE) is contained in the regulatory region of these cell types. Liu et al. (2006) hypothesized that sera taken from African American subjects with low $25(OH)D$ would be inefficient in supporting cathelicidin mRNA induction. This is indeed what they found. This lack of mRNA induction was reversed through the addition of $25(OH)D$ to those samples with low $25(OH)D$ levels. Thus, in this series of experiments, the addition of $25(OH)D_3$ restored the ability of sera from African American individuals to support TLR2/1L mediated induction of cathelicidin mRNA.

---

[10] The toll-like receptors (TLRs) are an extended family of host, noncatalytic transmembrane patterns-recognition receptors that interact with specific pathogen-specific membrane patterns called PAMPs. PAMPs are shed as infectious agents, such as tuberculosis, and trigger the innate immune system in the host—as we have just described.

The data support the premise that there is a link between toll-like receptors and vitamin D–mediated innate immunity, and it further suggests that differences in the ability of human populations to produce vitamin D may contribute to susceptibility to microbial infection and other long latency diseases. These exciting findings support the premise that vitamin D—through the actions of 25(OH)D activate monocytes and macrophages through innate immune system pathways. This landmark study paved the way for our understanding of vitamin D's important role in a diverse array of inflammatory diseases, such as multiple sclerosis, rheumatoid arthritis, cancers, diabetes, cardiovascular disease, and infection.

Not limited to the innate immune system, there is evidence to suggest that vitamin D also exerts an effect on the adaptive immune system that involves activation of T and B lymphocytes. As Bikle et al. stated so succinctly:

> *Contrary to the role of locally produced 1,25(OH)$_2$D to promote the innate immune response, the hormone exerts a generalized dampening effect on lymphocyte function. With respect to B cells, 1,25(OH)$_2$D suppresses proliferation and immunoglobulin production and retards the differentiation of B-lymphocyte precursors to mature plasma cells. With regard to T cells, 1,25(OH)$_2$D acting through the VDR, inhibits the proliferation of uncommitted T$_H$ (helper) cells…the hormone [also] promotes the proliferation of immunosuppressive regulatory T cells, so called T$_{reg}$S, and promotes their accumulation at sites of inflammation.…In fact, it is this generalized ability of 1,25(OH)$_2$D to quell the adaptive immune response, which has prompted the use of the hormone and its analogs in the adjuvant treatment of autoimmune and neoplastic disorders"* (Bikle et al., 2008, p. 145-146).

The findings in the laboratory explain the significant association between vitamin D and

(1) Various autoimmune diseases, such as:
a. Lupus (Kamen et al., 2006).
b. Multiple sclerosis (Kieseier, Giovannoni, & Hartung, 1999; Hayes, 2000; Munger et al., 2004; Chaudhuri, 2005; Ponsonby, Lucas, & vanderMei, 2005; Willer et al.,

2005; Munger et al., 2006; Arnson, Amital, & Shoenfeld, 2007; Kimball, Ursell, O'Connor, & Vieth, 2007).

    c.   Rheumatoid arthritis (Merlino et al., 2004; Ponsonby et al., 2005; Cutolo, Otsa, Uprus, Paolino, & Seriolo, 2007).

    d.   Diabetes—both Type 1 (Boucher, 1995; The EURODIAB Substudy 2 Study Group, 1999; Hypponen et al., 2001; Shehadeh, Shamir, Berant, & Etzioni, 2001; Holick, 2004; Hypponen, 2004; Caicedo, Li, Atkinson, Schatz, & Neu, 2005; Harris, 2005; Ponsonby et al., 2005) and Type-2 (Ford, Ajani, McGuire, & Liu, 2005; Liu et al., 2005; Pittas, Lau, Hu, & Dawson-Hughes, 2007).

(2) Certain cancers, such as:

    a.   Colon (Garland et al., 1989; Tseng, Breslow, Graubard, & Ziegler, 2005; Giovannucci, 2007; Hu et al., 2007; Wu et al., 2007).

    b.   Breast (Eisman et al., 1981; Sher et al., 1981; Garland, Garland, Gorham, & Young, 1990; Garland et al., 2007; Lin et al., 2007; Mordan-McCombs, Valrance, Zinser, Tenniswood, & Welsh, 2007; Robien, Cutler, & Lazovich, 2007; Rohan, 2007; Freedman et al., 2008).

    c.   Prostate (Rao, 2002; Platz, Leitzmann, Hollis, Willett, & Giovannucci, 2004; Tseng et al., 2005; Giovannucci et al., 2006; Feldman, Krishnan, Moreno, Swami, Peehl, & Srinivas, 2007; Giovannucci, 2007; Ingles, 2007; Mikhak et al., 2007; Mordan-McCombs et al., 2007; Weigel, 2007; Freedman et al., 2008).

(3) Other inflammatory diseases, such as cardiovascular disease and hypertension (Giovannucci et al., 2008; Wang et al., 2008).

This is an exciting example of translational research at its best—linking disease states with a single modifier. It is true that the modifier—in this case, vitamin D—is not a simple modifier, but its singular ability to impact on immune function is in evidence. Such considerations must be taken into account when considering the implications of vitamin D sufficiency or deficiency, and both their short-term and long-term sequelae.

9. DEFINING VITAMIN D SUFFICIENCY

BY CAROL L. WAGNER, M.D., AND BRUCE W. HOLLIS, PH.D.

What Constitutes Sufficiency? Where Do We Start?

For starters, one has to understand the nomenclature of nutritional sciences set forth by the Institute of Medicine (Food & Nutrition Board, 1997). There is a distinction between dietary recommended intake (DRI) and Adequate Intake (AI). DRI replaced the old nomenclature of Recommended Dietary Allowance, or RDA, and refers to the dietary intake level that is sufficient to meet the nutrient requirements of nearly all (>97%) healthy individuals in a particular life stage and gender group. In comparison, the Adequate Intake or AI refers to a recommended intake value based on observed or experimentally determined approximations or estimates of nutrient intake by a group (or groups) of healthy people that are assumed to be adequate and is used when a DRI/RDA cannot be determined. Thus, because of the paucity of data at the last Institute of Medicine's discussion about vitamin D requirements across the lifespan, a DRI does not exist for vitamin D today; rather, there are only recommendations made concerning the AI for vitamin D (Institute of Medicine, 1990).

There are also such terms as Estimated Average Requirement, which is the nutrient intake estimated to meet the requirement defined by a specified indicator of adequacy in 50% of an age- and gender-specific group. Lastly, the Tolerable Upper Intake Level (UL) is the highest level of daily nutrient intake that is likely to pose no risk of adverse health effects for almost all of the individuals in the general population. As intake increases above the UL, the risk of adverse effects increases.

The second point that needs to be discussed is what marker do you use to measure vitamin D status? Is it circulating 25(OH)D, $1,25(OH)_2D$, vitamin D itself, or a combination? In truth, the best indicator is the circulating concentration of 25(OH)D, as it represents the cumulative effects of exposure to sunlight and dietary intake of vitamin D (Haddad & Hahn, 1973; Lund & Sorensen, 1979; Holick, 1995b; Hollis, 2005). As we learned in **Section 7**, liver vitamin D-25-hydroxylase is regulated by vitamin D and its metabolites, and therefore, the increase in circulating concentration of 25(OH)D after exposure to sunlight or ingestion of vitamin D is relatively modest compared with cumulative production or intake of vitamin D (Holick & Clark, 1978). Because the appearance in the blood of vitamin D itself is short-lived, as it is either stored in the fat or metabolized in the liver (Mawer, Backhouse, Holman, Lumb, & Stanbury, 1972), it is more vulnerable to daily fluctuations in sunlight exposure or vitamin D intake, and thus, is not a good indicator of your overall vitamin D status. Similarly, 1,25(OH)$_2$D, with its short half-life and the body's tendency to maintain levels even in the face of extreme substrate deficiency, is not a good indicator of your overall vitamin D status. In comparison, 25(OH)D, with its much longer half-life in the human circulation of approximately 10 days to 3 weeks (Mawer, Schaefer, Lumb, & Stanbury, 1971; Mawer et al., 1972; Vicchio et al., 1993) and its greater (2-5 times more) activity than giving vitamin D itself in curing rickets and in inducing intestinal calcium absorption and mobilization of calcium from bones in rats, is the better index to measure.

At the same time as the knowledge of the role of vitamin D in health has expanded, the definition of healthy vitamin D status has shifted as studies have shown ill-effects at low vitamin D levels previously considered within the normal range (Sherman et al., 1990; Gloth, Tobin, Sherman, & Hollis, 1991; Gloth, Gundberg, Hollis, Haddad, & Tobin, 1995; Heaney, Dowell, Hale, & Bendich, 2003; Heaney, Davies, Chen, Holick, & Barger-Lux, 2003; Vieth, Ladak, & Walfish, 2003; Bischoff-Ferrari, Dietrich, Orav, & Dawson-Hughes, 2004; Chiu, Chu, Go, & Soad, 2004; Hollis, 2005; Hollis, Wagner, Kratz, Sluss, & Lewandrowski, 2005; Whiting & Calvo, 2005; Holick, 2007a; Hollis, 2007; Vieth et al., 2007; Hollis, 2009). Studies now almost 40 years ago, evaluating vitamin D status, measured 25(OH)D levels in populations that appeared clinically healthy without the stigmata of rickets or bony diseases. The subjects chosen for the studies were considered healthy in vitamin D status because they represented the general population and not because of known vitamin D sufficiency. The data were then plotted, using a Gaussian distribution to define "normal" (Haddad & Chyu, 1971;

Haddad & Stamp, 1974). These studies became the basis for definition of the lower limit of normal vitamin D status as 10-15 ng/mL (Institute of Medicine, 1990).

As will be discussed later, more recent studies have evaluated the *effect* of vitamin D deficiency and have defined "normal" as the absence of markers of insufficient vitamin D status. For example, many studies have shown a significant, inverse relationship between circulating 25(OH)D and parathyroid hormone (PTH), with a vitamin D level < 32 ng/ml (80 nmol/L) inducing secondary hyperparathyroidism (Sherman et al., 1990; Gloth et al., 1991; Vieth et al., 2003; Harkness & Cromer, 2005a, b). To truly appreciate these finer points, it is important to review how we got to this perspective.

Another Lesson from History

Another excellent review by Dr. Reinhold Vieth (Vieth, 1999) addresses the history of how the requirements for vitamin D were determined in the general adult population. In summary, before 1997, the AI for vitamin D in infants and children was 10 µg (400 IU) (National Academy of Sciences,1989). As mentioned earlier in **Sections 4 and 5**, the scientific basis for this dose was that it approximated what was in a teaspoon of cod-liver oil and had long been considered safe and effective in preventing rickets (Park, 1940). This has proven to be correct and has been the basis for prescribing 400 IU vitamin D per day to children (Rajakumar, 2003; Cannell et al., 2008). Unfortunately, the basis for adult vitamin D recommendations is even less well defined.

Now more than forty years ago, an expert committee on vitamin D could provide only anecdotal support for what it referred to as "the hypothesis of a small requirement" for vitamin D in adults, and recommended one-half the infant dose, just to ensure that adults obtain some from the diet (Blumberg et al., 1963). In England, an adult requirement of only 2.5 µg (100 IU)/day was substantiated on the basis of seven adult women with severe nutritional osteomalacia whose bones showed a response when given this amount (Smith & Dent, 1969). As pediatricians, we prescribe medications to children on a per kilogram basis; thus, 400 IU prescribed to a 3 kg neonate is approximately 133 IU per kg. Compare this to an adult who weighs 60 kg, 70 kg, etc. The dose by simple mathematics becomes inconsequential. This aspect of vitamin D would not matter if one would ensure enough substrate—parent vitamin D compound could be supplied to the body through sunlight exposure. As we have seen, this is not the case in the 21st century for the vast majority.

Despite the simple mathematical view of vitamin D dosing on a per kilogram basis, the recommendation for the adult AI of 5 µg (200 IU)/day that was reconfirmed as a "generous allowance" in the 1989 version of American Recommended Intakes (National Academy of Sciences, 1989) continues today. As was mentioned earlier, the basis for these recommendations—studies in the literature, occurred *before* it was possible to measure the circulating level of 25(OH)D, the indicator of nutritional vitamin D status (Haddad & Stamp, 1974; Hollis, 1996). If one looks at the timeline of vitamin D characterization and the ability to measure circulating 25(OH)D, the earliest reliable laboratory assays were not available until the 1970's (Haddad & Chyu, 1971). Even if we had the ability to measure circulating 25(OH)D easily and consistently back then, it would not have changed recommendations because the concept that vitamin D could affect other systems besides calcium and bone metabolism was not appreciated until recently.

The Lowest Observed Adverse Effect Level (LOAEL) or Highest Tolerated Dose Without Toxicity

Equally important with respect to dietary vitamin D intakes involves the LOAEL. Because there was lack of evidence to support statements about the toxicity of moderate doses of vitamin D, caution prevailed. For instance, the statement in the 1989 U.S. Nutrition Guidelines states that five times the DRI for vitamin D may be harmful (National Academy of Sciences, 1989). These Guidelines, in turn, relate back to a 1963 expert committee report (Park, 1940), which then refers back to the primary reference, a 1938 report in which linear bone growth in infants was suppressed in those given 45-158 µg (1,800-6,300 IU) vitamin D/day (Jeans & Stearns, 1938). The study was not conducted in adults and, thus, does not form a scientific basis for a safe upper limit in adults.

The same applies to the statement in the 1987 Council Report for the American Medical Association that "…dosages of 10,000 IU/day for several months have resulted in marked disturbances in calcium metabolism with hypercalcemia, hyperphosphatemia, hypertension, anorexia, nausea, vomiting, weakness, polyuria, polydipsia, azotemia, nephrolithiasis, ectopic calcification, renal failure, and, in some cases—death" (Council on Scientific Affairs, 1987, p. 1934-1935). Two references were cited to substantiate this. One was a review article about vitamins in general, which gave no evidence for and cited no other reference to its claim of toxicity at vitamin D doses as low as 250 µg (10,000 IU/day) (Woolliscroft, 1983). The other paper cited in the report dealt with 10 patients with vitamin D toxicity reported in 1948, for whom the vitamin D dose was actually 3,750-15,000 µg (150,000 – 600,000 IU)/day (Howard & Meyer, 1948); of note, all patients recovered.

In the 1990 Institute of Medicine publication, *Nutrition During Pregnancy*, these points were reiterated. The issue of poorly substantiated claims of toxicity extends even to the most recent revision for vitamin D intakes published by the National Academy of Sciences (Standing Committee Dietary Reference Intakes, 1997). One cannot blame the agencies and academies for their cautious point of view. There was little data—compared to the current plethora of data, these scientists could only quote less than ideal studies and the "exuberance" during which vitamin D was prescribed in post-World War II era in Great Britain when millions of international units of vitamin D were inadvertently, and sometimes advertently, given. Evidence-based medicine was born out of such uncontrolled trials that had little substantiated data.

Speaking of substantiated data, up until the recent independent toxicity studies of Vieth et al. (Vieth, 1999; Vieth, Chan, & MacFarlane, 2001) and Heaney et al. (Heaney, Davies, et al., 2003), the only study that could be cited to address the question of critical endpoint doses for vitamin D (potential adverse effect level) was a study by Narang et al. (Narang, Gupta, Jain, & Aaronson, 1984). The basis for the current no observed adverse effect level (NOAEL) of 50 µg (2,000 IU)/day is that Narang et al. reported a mean serum calcium concentration >11 mg/dL in the 6 "normal" subjects given 95 µg (3,800 IU) vitamin D/day; this intake became the lowest observed adverse effect level (LOAEL). The next lowest test dose used by Narang et al. (1984) was 60 µg (2,400 IU)/day, with 20% less as the safety margin, becoming the NOAEL. Narang et al. reported only serum electrolyte changes; the doses of vitamin D were not verified and circulating 25(OH)D levels were not reported.

Recent reports by Vieth et al. (Vieth, Chan, et al., 2001) and Heaney et al. (Heaney, Davies, et al., 2003) call into question the issue of vitamin D toxicity above 2000 IU per day. As originally stated by Vieth (1999), we have yet to find published evidence of toxicity in adults from an intake of 250 μg (10,000 IU)/day that is verified by the circulating 25(OH)D concentration. The LOAEL and NOAEL for vitamin D in the adult human have been established with insufficient scientific evidence, and thus require correction through sound scientific studies, many of which are ongoing.

The Adequate Intake (AI) for Infants, Children, and Adults on a Per Kilogram Basis

As we mentioned earlier in this section, the question that has intrigued our group for years is the following: how is it possible that the AI for vitamin D is the same for a 1-kg premature human infant, a 3.5-kg term infant, and a 90-kg adult? The recommendation for all of these subjects is 200-400 IU (5-10 μg)/day! To answer this question, it is necessary to ascertain the effect of a 400 IU daily intake of vitamin D on circulating 25(OH)D levels in infants and adults. We published the results of a study in infants more than 19 years ago (Pittard, Geddes, Hulsey, & Hollis, 1991). In this study, term (weight 3.4 ± 0.4 kg) and preterm (1.3 ± 0.2 kg) infants were supplemented with 400 IU (10 μg) vitamin D/day for 4 months. Circulating 25(OH)D (ng/mL), the nutritional indicator of vitamin D status, increased during this period in the term (11 ± 9 to 26 ± 12 ng/mL) and preterm (11 ± 5 to 51 ± 19 ng/mL) infants. These are significant increases that resulted in levels >20 ng/mL. Our recent interim analysis of infants randomized to the control group of our ongoing lactation study as a safety check reconfirms that 400 IU vitamin D/day will substantially increase infant circulating 25(OH)D levels (Wagner et al., 2010 (see **Section 11** for more detail). Thus, a daily dose of 400 IU (10 μg) vitamin D appears to be effective in raising the vitamin D nutritional status to the accepted normal range for infants (15-80 ng/mL).

What does a 400 IU daily dose for an extended time (months), however, do for an adult? The answer is little or nothing. Circulating 25(OH)D levels usually remain unchanged or decline. This was first demonstrated in both adolescent girls and young women (Lehtonen-Veromaa et al., 1999; Vieth, Cole, Hawker, Trang, & Rubin, 2001). Yet, at this dose (10 µg/day) in an adult, circulating 25(OH)D levels usually remain unchanged or decline. In another study involving adult submariners, even 600 IU/day of vitamin D *did not* maintain circulating 25(OH)D (Holick, 1994). In our prior two pilot lactation studies, 400 IU vitamin D/day were irrelevant in increasing maternal circulating 25(OH)D levels at 1 month baseline (Hollis & Wagner, 2004b; Wagner et al., 2006) and in the control group of our second pilot study (Wagner et al., 2006) (see **Section 12** for more detail). The question remains then, what level of vitamin D intake is required to maintain or preferably increase nutritional vitamin D status in the adult and in the adult who is pregnant or lactating?

This is a complex scientific question, yet recent well-controlled studies have provided some provisional answers (Vieth, Chan, et al., 2001; Heaney, Davies, et al., 2003). First, what is the "normal" circulating level of 25(OH)D in the adult population? Prior to 2004, data taken from the Mayo Medical Labs in Rochester, Minnesota, listed the normal, total circulating 25(OH)D range to be 15-80 ng/mL (37.5-200 nmol/L) (Favus, 1999). Since that time, the lower limit has been increased to 25 ng/mL (62.5 nmol/L) (Hurley & Singh, 2006). This revised range is in accordance with what we find in our laboratory; however, the level of circulating 25(OH)D is dependent on season and latitude, as evidenced by the reference ranges (Hollis et al., 1993). In sun-rich environments, circulating 25(OH)D is in the range of 54-90 ng/mL (Haddad & Kyung, 1971; Haddock et al., 1982; Matsuoka, Wortsman, Hanifan, et al., 1988), and in our experience, we have not found toxicity with circulating 25(OH)D levels that reached up to 100 ng/mL.

As we have discussed before, most studies prior to the 1990s concentrated on how much vitamin D is required to avoid deficiency as defined by the development of rickets or osteoporosis. Available evidence in which circulating intact PTH and 25(OH)D were measured in adult patients indicates that 2° hyperparathyroidism occurs when serum 25(OH)D values fall below the range of 15-20 ng/mL (Lips et al., 1988; Gloth et al., 1991; Gloth et al., 1995). A recent report by Vieth et al. (2003) demonstrates that maximal suppression of PTH by circulating 25(OH)D occurs at >80 nmol/L (32 ng/mL) 25(OH)D. Heaney et al. (Heaney, Dowell, et al., 2003) have demonstrated in normal adults that intestinal calcium absorptive performance is reduced in individuals who exhibit circulating 25(OH)D levels of 20 ng/mL (50 nmol/L) compared to subjects with circulating levels >32 ng/mL (80 nmol/L). They concluded that individuals with circulating 25(OH)D levels at the low end of the current reference range may not be getting the full benefit from their calcium intake. Recent, additional retrospective and interventional studies suggest that circulating 25(OH)D needs to exceed 80 nmol/L to maximize skeletal integrity (Bischoff-Ferrari et al., 2004; Meier, Woitge, Witte, Lemmer, & Seibel, 2004).

Normative Adult Data in a Sun-Rich Environment

Humans evolved thousands of years ago in an environment that had significant sunlight exposure, generating in excess of 20,000 IU (500 μg) vitamin D/day from that exposure. In fact, a half hour in the summer sun between 10 a.m. and 2 p.m. in a bathing suit (approximately 3 times the minimal erythemal dose exposure) will initiate the release of approximately 50,000 IU (1.25 mg) vitamin D into the circulation within 24 hours of exposure in a Caucasian individual (Adams, Clements, Parrish, & Holick, 1982). An African American individual will require up to 5 times the solar exposure to achieve the same response (Clemens et al., 1982; Matsuoka et al., 1991). In Caucasians who have a deep tan because of the melanin deposition in the skin, the response will be cut approximately in half, so only 20,000-30,000 IU (500-750 μg) of vitamin D will be liberated (Matsuoka et al., 1990a). Finally, if you wear clothing or total body sunscreen, the cutaneous release of vitamin D will be completely blunted (Matsuoka, Wortsman, Hanifan, et al., 1988; Matsuoka et al., 1989; Matsuoka et al., 1990b; Matsuoka et al., 1992). So, in light of the above facts, the 200-400 IU/day (5-10 μg) vitamin D/ day recommendation in the adult seems woefully inadequate to maintain normal circulating levels of vitamin D in adults with minimal solar exposure.

As Defined by Levels of 25(OH)D in the Sun-Replete Adult, How Much Vitamin D Intake Is Required to Sustain an Adequate Nutritional Vitamin D Status?

For Caucasians who experience significant body solar exposure on a routine basis, this is not an important question. As a population, however, our unprotected exposure to the sun is declining rapidly (fueled by the realistic fear of skin cancer, whose incidence continues to rise, and premature aging). For individuals with darker pigmentation, the answer is more complicated: The darker pigmentation of the African American population is a powerful natural sunscreen, which given the constraints of modern-day and urban dwelling, adversely affects cutaneous vitamin D synthesis.

The first study to address this topic was published by Vieth et al. in 2001. In this study, the investigators supplemented normal adults daily with either 25 µg (1,000 IU) or 100 µg (4,000 IU) of vitamin D for a period of 5 months. The circulating 25(OH)D (ng/mL) increased from 16.3 ± 6.2 to 27.5 ± 6.8 and 18.7 ± 6.0 to 38.6 ± 5.8 in the 1,000 and 4,000 IU groups, respectively. It is important to note that there was not a single adverse event related to vitamin D and not one episode of hypercalciuria observed in the 60 subjects enrolled in the study.

In an even more detailed report, Heaney et al. (Heaney, Davies, et al., 2003) studied 67 men divided into four groups who were randomized to receive 0 IU (0µg) 200 IU (5 µg), 1000 IU (25 µg), 5000 IU (125 µg), or 10,000 IU (250 µg) vitamin D/day for a period of 5 months. The 200 IU/day group failed to maintain circulating 25(OH)D levels during the study period. The remaining three groups responded in a dose-response fashion with respect to rises in circulating 25(OH)D levels. From these data, using regression analysis, it has become possible to calculate a response of circulating 25(OH)D from a given oral intake of vitamin D. The data reveal that for every 1 µg (40 IU) of vitamin D intake, circulating 25(OH)D rises by 0.28 ng/mL (or 0.7 nmol/L) over 5 months on a given supplemental regimen. It should be noted that a steady-state appears to be achieved after approximately 90 days on each dose tested (Vieth, Chan, et al., 2001; Heaney, Davies, et al., 2003). Thus, a 400 IU (10 µg), 1000 IU (25 µg), 4000 IU (100 µg), or 10,000 IU (250 µg) daily dose for a period of 5 months will result in theoretical circulating increases of 2.8, 7.0, 28, and 70 ng/mL 25(OH)D, respectively, all of which remain in the normal circulating level range according to the reference range data (Favus, 1999). In the Heaney study, not one case of hypercalcemia or hypercalciuria was observed (Heaney, Davies, et al., 2003).

The Final Frontier: Defining Normal Nutritional Vitamin D Status

We come back to this question as the conclusion and summation of this section. What is the adequate intake for vitamin D in the neonate, the infant, the young child, the 10-year-old, the adolescent, the adult, and the adult who is pregnant or lactating in order to achieve optimal circulating concentrations of 25(OH)D? Before that question can be answered, the optimal concentration of circulating 25(OH)D needs to be determined across the lifespan and based on body mass. Most studies have concentrated on how much vitamin D is required to avoid deficiency as manifested by bony changes, such as rickets and osteopenia (Gartner et al., 2003; Hollis, 2005; Hollis, 2009).

Available evidence in which circulating intact PTH and 25(OH)D measured in adult patients indicates that secondary hyperparathyroidism occurs when serum 25(OH)D values fall below a certain range that traditionally was below the range of 15-20 ng/mL (Lips et al., 1988; Gloth et al., 1991; Gloth et al., 1995). Some think it really is 30-32 ng/mL (80 nmol/L) (Dawson-Hughes et al., 2005; Hollis et al., 2007; Vieth et al., 2007). Supporting this higher inflection point between 25(OH)D and PTH, Vieth et al. (2003) found maximal suppression of PTH by circulating 25(OH)D in their cohort at >80 nmol/L (32 ng/mL) 25(OH)D. This premise is supported by other data: Heaney et al. (Heaney, Dowell, et al., 2003) demonstrated in normal adults that intestinal calcium absorption was reduced in individuals who exhibited circulating 25(OH)D levels of 20 ng/mL compared to subjects with circulating levels >32 ng/mL. The authors concluded that individuals with circulating 25(OH)D levels at the low end of the current reference range may not be getting the full benefit from their calcium intake. Recent, additional retrospective and interventional studies suggest that circulating 25(OH)D needs to exceed 80 nmol/L to maximize skeletal integrity (Bischoff-Ferrari et al., 2004; Meier et al., 2004). Some of this data, as well as additional studies, have been summarized in recent reviews regarding the optimization of circulating 25(OH)D levels (Hollis, 2005; Vieth et al., 2007; Bikle et al., 2008, Vieth, 2009a; Vieth, 2009b).

If we are to answer the question fully—of what optimal vitamin D status is across the lifespan, we must encourage ourselves as consumers and as healthcare professionals to "broaden our horizon" and think of vitamin D in more global terms. We must think of vitamin D as a multi-functional hormonal system that affects not only calcium and bone metabolism, but also which affects both the adaptive and innate immune systems, all of which have profound implications on one's overall health status. When we think in these terms, it is readily apparent that the current reference ranges for circulating 25(OH)D are set too low, and that our "target" range of values should be those we find in individuals who live outdoors in a sun-rich environment (Haddad & Chyu, 1971; Haddock et al, 1982; Matsuoka, Wortsman, Hanifan, et al. 1988).

10. Vitamin D Requirements during Pregnancy

By Carol L. Wagner, M.D., and Bruce W. Hollis, Ph.D.

Maternal Link to Fetal and Early Infant Vitamin D Status

At no other time than during pregnancy and lactation is the mother directly responsible for the growth and development of her fetus and infant. Maternal well-being and nutritional status are linked with that of her fetus and breastfeeding infant. Most nutrients in the mother are transferred to the fetus at the expense of the mother. During extreme deficiencies, both the mother and her fetus are affected, including during vitamin D deficiency where the fetal condition parallels the maternal condition. Until recently, little was known about the vitamin D requirements of the pregnant and lactating woman. Even today, despite expanding knowledge about vitamin D's role in maintaining health in a whole host of areas, studies continue to report extensive vitamin D insufficiency and deficiency among pregnant and lactating women and their infants, particularly those with darker pigmentation, living at higher latitudes, and who have little sunlight exposure (Hollis & Wagner 2004a; Hollis, 2007; Johnson D, Wagner, et al, 2010, in press).

We have little consensus about the vitamin D requirements of women during these vulnerable periods. The appropriate dose of vitamin D during pregnancy and lactation is unknown, although it appears to be far greater than the current Adequate Intake (AI) of 200-400 IU/d (5-10 µg/d) (Institute of Medicine, 1990a). During the past 7 years, studies specifically reevaluating the AI during pregnancy (www.clinicaltrials.gov #NCT00292591, #NCT00412087) and lactation [2 prior studies (Hollis & Wagner, 2004b; Wagner et al., 2006) and one ongoing #NCT00412074] were initiated by our group; and others (www.clinicaltrials.gov: Copenhangen Asthma Study #NCT00856947; Dawodu United Arab of Emirates' study #NCT00610688), with the list of new clinical trials growing each month. This reassessment is critical since the current recommendations result in a high degree of vitamin D-deficiency, especially in the African-American and Hispanic populations and in those with darker skin pigmentation or decreased sunlight exposure (Nesby-O'Dell et al. 2002).

This avenue of research began in the late 1990s in the normal adult population (Vieth, Chan et al. 2001; Heaney, Davies et al. 2003), which paved the way for later clinical trials in more vulnerable populations, such as pregnant and lactating women and their children. The history of vitamin D dietary requirements and recommendations, and the issues of toxicity and hypervitaminosis D were discussed in earlier sections (**Sections 3-7**). Suffice it to say that while we know vastly more about vitamin D, for all intents and purposes until the last year or so, we knew little more in terms of "best practice" and how to advise the pregnant woman about vitamin D than half a century ago, and we still await the results of ongoing clinical trials to decipher what the actual requirements of vitamin D are for both the lactating mother and her infant. It has taken rigorous study of the pregnant and lactating woman's vitamin D status and careful oversight of supplementation trials to come to where we are today. We still have much more to discover, but we are no longer "stuck" in 20th century rhetoric. The tools of the 21st century have provided us with sophisticated measures that translate into better safety parameters and enhanced understanding of vitamin D during pregnancy.

With that being said, in the next several sections of **Section 10**, we will review what is known about maternal metabolism of vitamin D during pregnancy, about placental and fetal metabolism, and how sufficiency can or cannot be achieved during pregnancy. We then review the implications of maternal status and its potential effect during early infancy and later life, with many questions still unanswered in **Section 11**. In **Section 12**, the discussion continues with a focus on the vitamin D requirements of the mother-infant dyad during breastfeeding, with an emphasis on the vitamin D content of human milk and how that content and transfer to the recipient infant may be influenced. First, let us start at the beginning—pregnancy and the fetal condition as it relates to vitamin D.

Vitamin D During Pregnancy—Why Is It important?

Since the 1920s, it has been known that maternal vitamin D concentration largely determines the vitamin D status of the developing fetus and neonate (Park 1923; Hess, 1929; Hillman & Haddad 1974). Vitamin D sufficiency is linked with bone mineralization and calcium homeostasis, important for the pregnant woman as well as the developing fetus. Profound vitamin D deficiency is linked with both maternal and neonatal hypocalcemia, as vitamin D is intricately associated with calcium absorption in the GI tract and reabsorption from the renal tubules.[11] It follows that if a woman is vitamin D deficient during her pregnancy, then her fetus will be developing in a low vitamin D state and will be at significant risk of vitamin D deficiency. Despite this observation, the systematic reviews by the Institute of Medicine in 1997 (Standing Committee Dietary Reference Intakes, 1997) and a Cochrane Review in 2002 (Mahomed & Gulmezoglu, 2002) concluded that little data existed regarding maternal vitamin D supplementation during pregnancy.

As we have already discussed, adult vitamin D deficiency is widespread; recent data indicate that an ideal level for total circulating 25(OH)D is at concentrations of at least 32 ng/mL (80 nmol/L) and preferably above 40 ng/mL or 100 nmol/L (Holick, 2007b). Levels between 20-32 ng/mL (50-80 nmol/L) are considered insufficiency (Johnson, Wagner, et al., 2010). The first report of widespread vitamin D deficiency in women of childbearing age in the U.S. came from the CDC NHANES III report revealing that 42% of African American women had 25(OH)D levels below serum concentrations of 15 ng/mL or 37.5 nmol/L (Nesby-O'Dell et al., 2002), and more recent data in a large cohort in South Carolina, with deficiency defined as 25(OH)D level below 20 ng/mL, suggests this prevalence is around 75% (Wagner, Johnson, et al., 2008). A long-standing unawareness of the short and long-term health consequences of vitamin D insufficiency has led to widespread insufficiencies in most populations.

A recent focus on fetal origin of adult disease has led to investigation of the exposure to vitamin D insufficiency during fetal development and its relationship to later disease processes (McGrath, 1999; McGrath, Feton, & Eyles, 2001; McGrath, Selten, & Chant, 2002; Brown, Bianco, McGrath, & Eyles, 2003; Eyles, Brown,

MacKay-Sim, McGrath, & Feron, 2003; Burne, Becker, et al., 2004; Burne, Feron, et al., 2004; Ko, Burkert, McGrath, & Eyles, 2004; Hollis, 2005; Kesby, Burne, McGrath, & Eyles, 2006; Cui, McGrath, Burne, Mackay-Sim, & Eyles, 2007; Hathcock, Shao, Vieth, & Heaney, 2007; Hollick, 2007a; O'Loan et al., 2007; Vieth et al., 2007, Vieth, 2009a). Such epidemiological data point to a relationship between schizophrenia and seasonal and geographic characteristics of the offspring who later develop the disease. These findings have been supported by studies using the rat model of vitamin D deficiency and measuring the effects on brain architecture and function. There was one report of long-term effects of maternal/ neonatal vitamin D status and later bone mass at 9 years (Javaid et al., 2006).

Because vitamin D status has not been a consistent concern during pregnancy, long-term data are sparse. The few studies that have been conducted have focused more on the neonatal effects of vitamin D during pregnancy, rather than the long-latency and later potential health effects. With severe maternal vitamin D deficiency, the fetus may rarely develop rickets *in utero* and manifest this deficiency at birth (Hatun et al., 2005; Schnadower, Agarwal, Oberfield, Fennoy, & Pusic, 2006). Supplementation with 400 IU vitamin D/day during the last trimester of pregnancy has minimal effect on circulating 25(OH)D concentrations in the mother and her infant at term (Cockburn et al., 1980). It stands to reason, then, that an unsupplemented infant born to a vitamin D-deficient mother will reach a state of deficiency more quickly than an infant whose mother was replete during pregnancy (Hollis & Wagner, 2004a).

But, and this is the truly million dollar question, if we have adequate information for at least the past two decades to show that 400 IU vitamin D/day is inadequate to prevent vitamin D deficiency *in the vast majority of pregnant women*, then why we are not giving higher supplementation doses? The answer lies in the history and the appropriate fear that higher doses of vitamin D are teratogenic. Until more recent times, the deleterious effects of vitamin D deficiency beyond calcium and bone metabolism were not appreciated, and if one looks to just bone metabolism and calcium homeostasis, it was felt by many learned individuals that the risk

---

[11] For a superb review of the effect of vitamin D on fetal and maternal calcium homeostasis, we refer you to the following: Kovacs, C. S. (2008). "Vitamin D in pregnancy and lactation: maternal, fetal, and neonatal outcomes from human and animal studies." Am J Clin Nutr 88(2): 520S-528.

of higher dose vitamin D supplementation, while unproven, was there and the benefit did not override the risk; that is, until recently. To understand from another angle how we got to this place of overwhelming deficiency in pregnant women, we must review the literature and findings that supported the premise of vitamin D's toxicity as it relates to the pregnant woman and her fetus.

Animal Models of Vitamin D Toxicity During Pregnancy: As mentioned previously in **Section 5**, animal models during pregnancy developed in the 1960-1970s were utilized to study vitamin D-induced SAS syndrome in humans (Latorre, 1961; Friedman & Roberts, 1966; Nebel & Ornoy, 1966; Ornoy & Nebel, 1967; Friedman & Mills, 1969; Ornoy, Nebel, & Menczel, 1969; Ornoy & Nebel, 1970; Nebel & Ornoy, 1971; Chan et al., 1979; Toda, Toda, & Kummerow, 1985; Fischer et al., 1991; Neiderhoffer, Bobryshev, Laftaud-Idjouadiene, Giummelly, & Atkinson, 1997; Norman, Moss, Sian, Gosling, & Powell, 2002). These animal models, almost without exception, focused on feeding or injecting rodents, rabbits, or pigs with toxic levels of vitamin D or administering the active form, $1,25(OH)_2D$, and assessing the biological consequences. The results arising from vitamin D-induced hypercalcemia were real, definable, and devastating extra-skeletal calcifications of the aorta (a defect not observed in Williams Syndrome) and other tissues, usually followed by death. In most of these studies, animals received 200,000-300,000 IU (5,000-7,500 μg)/kg body weight of vitamin D to elicit these horrendous effects. As noted earlier, an equivalent dose to a 60-kg human would be 15,000,000 IU (375,000 μg)/day. In fact, toxic levels of vitamin D have been used as rodenticide in the past, as an alternative to warfarin. To put this toxicity into human terms, in order to achieve the same results in humans, *millions* of units of vitamin D would have to be given.

Two relatively recent publications dealing with vitamin D supplementation during pregnancy and fetal cardiac abnormalities using animal models need to be addressed. The first of these articles was published in 1985 in the *Japanese Science Journal* (Toda et al., 1985). These investigators fed a total of 2 (*yes, it is a sample size of two*) pregnant pigs a different dose of vitamin D. One pig was fed an almost vitamin D-deficient diet, the other a diet with a relatively normal vitamin D content. The piglets from the low vitamin D mother exhibited borderline hypovitaminosis D (15 ng/mL circulating 25(OH)D), while piglets from the other sow possessed normal circulating levels of 25(OH)D. The authors attempted to relate normal circulating 25(OH)D in the piglets to coronary arterial lesions and made the inference that this could be the reason Americans have a high rate of coronary disease. This study lacked the power to detect any statistically significant differences.

Only one other study has been reported that attempts to repeat the results of the porcine study using a rat model (Norman et al., 2002). In this study, investigators fed pregnant rats the *hormonal* form of vitamin D, $1,25(OH)_2D_3$, directly. The intake of $1,25(OH)_2D_3$ by these pregnant rats was shown to influence rat aortic structure, function, and elastin content. These investigators collected the blood using EDTA, a calcium chelating agent, as an anticoagulant; as a consequence, circulating calcium could not even be measured! Thus, clinically significant hypervitaminosis D could not be demonstrated by the primary effect— hypercalcemia, invalidating the study. In addition, since the authors used the hormonal form of vitamin D—$1,25(OH)_2D_3$, this constitutes a pharmacological study, and in doing so, does not represent or recapitulate normal physiology in humans. That is to say, the hormonal form was given, bypassing the body's normal regulation of the conversion of 25(OH)D to $1,25(OH)_2D$. Thus, these animal studies have no bearing on normal human nutrition.

Animal Models of Vitamin D Deficiency During Pregnancy: Conversely, other studies to investigate the effects of vitamin D deficiency and how important adequate nutritional levels of vitamin D are to skeletal, cardiovascular, and neurodevelopment in experimental animals have been undertaken (Marie, Cancela, LeBoulch, & Miravet, 1986; Weishaar & Simpson, 1987; Weishaar, Kim, Saunders, & Simpson, 1990; Morris, Zhou, Hegsted, & Keenan, 1995; Eyles et al., 2003).

Perhaps the best-known and widely accepted effects of vitamin D are on the skeletal system, which have been easily replicated in animal models throughout the decades. Where thought and dogma are, studies follow, so it is not surprising, and certainly not unexpected, that adequate vitamin D is required for normal skeletal development. The importance of vitamin D to skeletal integrity has been demonstrated in a study involving rodents (Marie et al., 1986). This study revealed that hypovitaminosis D during pregnancy impaired endosteal bone formation, which resulted in trabecular bone loss, and concluded that vitamin D is indispensable for normal bone mineralization during the reproductive period in the rat.

When we move beyond skeletal development, however, there are those of you in the audience at large who become a bit uncomfortable. Extending vitamin D into the realm of other systems beyond bone seems a bit risky, a bit less certain, yet there is increasing evidence that vitamin D affects extraskeletal systems in both animal models and in humans. Weisler and Simpson demonstrated that lengthy periods of vitamin D-deficiency in rats are associated with profound changes in cardiovascular function, including increases in cardiac and vascular muscle contractile function (Weishaar & Simpson, 1987). These investigators later demonstrated by histological examination that ventricular muscles from vitamin D-deficient rats exhibited a significant increase in extracellular space (Weishaar et al., 1990). Morris et al. (1995) reported that low maternal consumption of vitamin D retarded metabolic and contractile development in the neonatal rat heart. They concluded that low maternal vitamin D intake results in a general, but significant slowing of neonatal cardiac development. It is interesting that more recent epidemiologic data show a strong link between vitamin D deficiency and cardiovascular risk factors, such as hypertension and congestive heart failure (Forman et al., 2007; Giovannucci, Liu, Hollis, & Rimm, 2008). It is possible that the seeds for such devastating adult diseases find their origins during fetal development, as it relates to vitamin D status and its immune function.

Moving from the cardiovascular system to the brain and central nervous system, there is evidence to suggest that vitamin D status impacts on that system as well. McGrath postulated, now more than a decade ago, that vitamin D could be involved in brain function and neurodevelopment (McGrath, 1999; McGrath, 2001). In 2003, McGrath and colleagues provided startling evidence with respect to the consequences of vitamin D-deficiency on the neurodevelopment of the fetus during pregnancy in a rat model (Eyles et al., 2003). Pups born to vitamin D-deficient mothers demonstrated cortex abnormalities, enlarged lateral ventricles, and more cell proliferation throughout the brain. Further, there were reductions in brain content of nerve growth factor and glial cell line-derived neurotrophic factor, and reduced expression of p75^{NTR}, the low-affinity neurotrophin receptor. These findings suggest that low maternal vitamin D has important ramifications for the developing brain. What remains to be shown is the human side of this process and its correlates. Stay tuned!

Human Studies Involving Pharmacologic Doses of Vitamin D During Pregnancy: Studies involving pregnant women with hypoparathyroidism before the advent of PTH replacement give us a glimpse into the range of tolerability of vitamin D in pregnant human subjects. In one study, the pregnant woman required the administration of 100,000 IU vitamin D (2.5 mg)/day throughout pregnancy in order to maintain serum calcium (Greer, Hollis, & Napoli, 1984). When tested, this neonate was found to have circulating 25(OH)D levels of 250 ng/mL at birth; yet, this infant was perfectly normal and healthy. This woman again became pregnant and subsequently delivered another normal, healthy term infant. Thus, there is no evidence in humans that even a 100,000 IU/day dose of vitamin D for extended periods during pregnancy results in any harmful effects. Similarly, pharmacological doses of 1,25(OH)$_2$D$_3$ given to a woman to treat hypocalcemic rickets during her pregnancy produced no ill effects on the developing fetus specifically evaluated for elfin facies and SAS (Marx, Swart, Hamstra, & Deluca, 1980). Lest someone misinterpret what is being said here, we are not suggesting that a pregnant woman in this day and age be given daily vitamin D at such extreme doses. That is unnecessary and could be potentially harmful. We include this case history because it helps us put into context the recommendation of taking 4,000 IU vitamin D/day, and why it makes sense physiologically, but also from the perspective of tolerability and risk of toxicity.

To support this premise still further, in another study, 15 pregnant women and their offspring treated with high dose vitamin D for hypoparathyroidism were followed closely for signs of fetal toxicity (Goodenday & Gordon, 1971). Because of the concern that high dose vitamin D (given in pharmacologic doses to treat hypoparathyroidism) could cause supravalvular aortic stenosis, the infants of these mothers underwent auscultation for significant murmurs or bruits over the entire chest, back, abdomen, and peripheral vessels. Further, the children were examined at ages ranging from 6 weeks to 16 years, with many of the children being examined several times over a 4-year period. None of the children had any of the craniofacial stigmata associated with infantile hypercalcemia, which is not surprising as we learned in **Section 5** that children who have such findings suffer from a genetic disorder called Williams Syndrome. Specifically, none had micrognathia or evidence of supravalvular aortic stenosis, pulmonary stenosis, or other detectable cardiovascular anomalies.

Going Beyond Animal Models: Do We Dare?

Given the fully-established and time-tested findings that vitamin D affects bone mineralization and skeletal development, it is not too much of a stretch of faith to entertain the premise that adequate nutritional vitamin D status during pregnancy is important for fetal skeletal development, tooth enamel formation, and perhaps general fetal growth and development (Brooke et al., 1980; Brooke, Butters, & Wood, 1981).

Evidence Continues to Accumulate: In a recent Canadian study by Mannion et al. (Mannion, Gray-Donald, & Koski, 2006), comparing growth parameters in newborn infants with the maternal intakes of milk and vitamin D during pregnancy, investigators found an association between vitamin D intake during pregnancy and birth weight, but not infant head circumference or length at birth. With every additional 40 IU of maternal vitamin D intake, there was an associated 11-g increase in birth weight.

Continuing along this line of evidence, Pawley and Bishop (Pawley & Bishop, 2004) studied 108 pregnant women and their offspring and found a significant association between umbilical cord 25(OH)D concentrations and head circumference at 3 and 6 months' postnatal age that persisted after adjusting for confounding factors; there was no association between maternal vitamin D status and birth weight or length. Maghbooli et al. found significantly wider posterior fontanelle diameter in neonates of mothers with vitamin D deficiency (as defined by a 25(OH)D level <34.9 nmmol/L or ~14 ng/mL) compared to neonates whose mothers were not deficient (Maghbooli et al., 2007). Others have found increased head circumferences of those infants whose mothers had vitamin D deficiency during the last trimester of pregnancy that correlates with the architectural changes in the vitamin D deficient pregnant rat model (Becker, Eyles, McGrath, & Grecksch, 2005; Feron et al., 2005; O'Loan et al., 2007). Others did not find an effect of maternal vitamin D status on fetal growth as measured by neonatal anthropomorphic measures (Prentice et al., 2009). Javaid et al., in their study of pregnant women in the U.K., found that higher maternal vitamin D status during pregnancy was associated with improved bone mineral content and bone mass in children at 9 years of age (Javaid et al., 2006).

What is the "take home message" here? It is most likely that vitamin D has some small effect on fetal growth, but the most significant effects are likely in the area of bone development, bone mineral content, and bone health later in life. It is even more likely that vitamin D has its most far-reaching and lasting effects on fetal immune development, but that is a speculation that will require continued and elegant study.

Effectiveness of Vitamin D Supplementation During Pregnancy

As mentioned earlier, the Cochrane Library issued a review of vitamin D supplementation during pregnancy (Mahomed & Gulmezoglu, 2002) in 2002, identifying seven studies on the topic (Brooke et al., 1980; Cockburn et al., 1980; Brooke et al., 1981; Marya, Rathee, Lata, & Mudgil, 1981; Maxwell, Ang, Brooke, & Brown, 1981; Ala-Houhala, 1985; Delvin, Salle, Glorieux, Adeleine, & David, 1986). However, only four reported clinical outcomes (Brooke et al., 1980; Cockburn et al., 1980; Brooke et al., 1981; Maxwell et al., 1981). The Cochrane Review concluded that there was not enough evidence to evaluate the requirements and effects of vitamin D supplementation during pregnancy. Presented below are five of the most clinically relevant studies offered by the Cochrane review plus three additional studies identified by our group:

Initial vitamin D supplementation studies during pregnancy were carried out in the early 1980s and extended into the 1990s:

(1) Brooke et al. (1980), studying British mothers of Asian descent, found a greater incidence of small-for-gestational age (SGA) infants born to mothers receiving placebo vs. mothers receiving 1,000 IU (25 µg) vitamin D_2/day during the final trimester of pregnancy.

Neonates in the placebo group also exhibited a greater fontanelle area as compared to the supplemented group. It must be noted that the placebo group in this study exhibited profound hypovitaminosis D. Of note, in this initial study, Brooke et al. (1980) described a dramatic rise, 50-60 ng/mL, in circulating 25(OH)D in both mother and neonate at term; however, given what we know about the pharmacokinetics of vitamin D, these results have not been reproducible (Mallet et al., 1986; Vieth, Chan, et al., 2001; Datta et al., 2002; Heaney, Davies, et al., 2003; Wagner et al., 2003) and are consistent with a dose response obtained by giving 10,000 IU (250 µg)/day vitamin D for a period of 3 months. There is also a possibility that the 25(OH)D assay methodology used in this study was flawed as was common during this early period. Despite the inconsistency with other study results, what is important is that those women in the placebo group were significantly vitamin D deficient.

(2) Follow-up studies by Brooke et al. (1981) were conducted with Asian mothers who again were provided with either placebo or 1,000 IU vitamin D_2/day during the last trimester of pregnancy. The follow-up data provided evidence that during the first year of life, the infants of the maternal placebo group gained less weight and had a lower rate of linear growth than did the infants of the maternal supplemented group.

(3) Cockburn et al. (1980) undertook a large vitamin D supplementation study involving over 1,000 pregnant subjects in England supplemented with 400 IU (10 µg) vitamin D_2/day from week 12 of gestation onward as compared to a placebo group. At this level of supplementation, serum levels of 25(OH)D in the supplemented group were only slightly higher as compared to the placebo group. A defect in dental enamel formation was observed in a higher proportion of the children at 3 years in the maternal placebo group.

(4) Maxwell et al. (1981) conducted a double-blind trial of administering vitamin D (1,000 IU/day) during the last trimester of pregnancy to Asian women living in London and found that supplemented

mothers had increased weight gain, and at term had significantly higher plasma levels of retinol-binding protein and thyroid-binding prealbumin, indicating better protein-calorie nutrition. Almost twice as many infants in the unsupplemented group weighed under 2,500 g at birth and had significantly lower retinol binding protein levels than that of infants of supplemented mothers.

(5) Delvin et al. (1986) randomized 40 pregnant women at 6 months of gestation to either placebo or 1000 IU vitamin D/day, with all deliveries later taking place during the month of June. All infants were singletons who were breastfed without postnatal vitamin D administration. There were no significant changes in maternal whole-blood or ionized calcium, PTH, or $1,25(OH)_2D$ concentrations between the groups; however, 25(OH)D concentrations increased after 45 and 90 days of supplementation (65 vs. 30 nmol/L at term). Infants born to control mothers had mean cord blood 25(OH)D levels of 17 nmol/L vs. 45 nmol/L in infants born to mothers in the treatment group; similarly, $1,25(OH)_2D$ levels were higher in the treatment vs. control group (147 vs. 95 pmol/L). There were no significant differences on total or ionized calcium, magnesium, or PTH. When the infants were studied again at 4 days of age, infants of mothers in the control group had the following lower laboratory indices when compared to the treatment group: lower mean total calcium, ionized calcium, 25(OH)D (12 vs 33 nmol/L), and $1,25(OH)_2D$ (140 vs. 225 mmol/L). Although PTH concentrations were higher among control mothers and their infants at all times, there was no statistically significant difference between the groups.

(6) Mallet et al. (1986) reported that supplementing vitamin D (1,000 IU [25 µg]/day) during the last trimester of pregnancy resulted in only a 5-6 ng/mL increase in circulating 25(OH)D levels in maternal and cord serum.

(7) Brunvard et al. (Brunvard, Quigstad, Urdal, & Haug, 1996) followed 30 pregnant Pakistani women free of chronic diseases who had uncomplicated pregnancies. Nearly all of the women exhibited

low (<15 ng/ml) circulating 25(OH)D, and nearly half exhibited secondary hyperparathyroidism. The maternal circulating PTH level was inversely related to the neonatal crown-heel length. These authors concluded that maternal vitamin D deficiency affected fetal growth through an effect on maternal calcium homeostasis.

(8) In the most recent study by Datta et al., 160 pregnant minority women in England were provided with 800-1,600 IU (20-40 μg) vitamin D for the duration of their pregnancy (Datta et al., 2002). Using modern assay technology for the determination of circulating 25(OH)D levels (Hollis et al., 1993), these investigators determined a rise in circulating 25(OH)D levels (ng/mL) from 5.8 ± 0.9 at the beginning of pregnancy to 11.2 ± 6.3 at term, following vitamin D supplementation consistent with ongoing, significant deficiency. Thus, mothers who were vitamin D deficient at the beginning of their pregnancy were still deficient at the end of their pregnancy after being supplemented with on 800-1,600 IU vitamin D/day throughout their pregnancy.

The above findings are precisely what the regression analysis from Heaney et al. (Heaney, Davies, et al., 2003) predicts would happen at the various vitamin D intakes. The results of these studies indicate that the Adequate Intake (AI) for vitamin D during pregnancy of 400 IU/day is grossly inadequate, especially with ethnic minorities. The Vieth (Vieth, Chan, et al., 2001) and Heaney (Heaney, Davies, et al., 2003) data, and our own data with pregnant (Wagner, Johnson, et al., 2010a; Wagner, McNeil, et al., 2010; Wagner, Johnson, et al., 2010b) and lactating women (Hollis & Wagner 2004b; Wagner, Hulsey, et al., 2006) suggest that doses well above 1,000 IU vitamin D/day are required to achieve a robust nutritional vitamin D status in pregnant women.

Mentioned earlier, recent work has demonstrated that in men and nonpregnant women taking oral vitamin D supplements, for every 40 IU of vitamin D ingested over a 4- to 5-month period, their circulating 25(OH)D will increase by approximately 0.70 nmol/L (Vieth, Chan, et al., 2001; Heaney, Davies, et al., 2003). As predicted by vitamin D kinetics, supplements of 1000 IU/day of vitamin D to pregnant women result in a 12.5 to 17.5 nmol/L increase in circulating 25(OH)D concentrations in both maternal and cord serum compared with nonsupplemented controls (Brooke et al., 1980; Brooke et al., 1981; Maxwell et al., 1981).

These findings were recently corroborated by our two randomized clinical trials involving vitamin D supplementation of pregnant women. The significance of these findings for those who care for the pediatric population is that when a woman who has vitamin D deficiency gives birth, her neonate also will be deficient. Preliminary analyses of the data indicate that 4000 IU vitamin D/day is an effective dose to achieve vitamin D sufficiency in the pregnant woman without safety issues related to that therapy (Wagner, Johnson, et al., 2010a; Wagner, McNeil, et al., 2010; Wagner, Johnson, et al. 2010b).

It is important to note that women with increased skin pigmentation or who have little exposure of their skin to sunlight are at a greater risk of vitamin D deficiency and may need additional vitamin D supplements, especially during pregnancy and lactation (Hollis & Wagner, 2004a). In a study by van der Meer et al., >50% of pregnant women with darker pigmentation in the Netherlands were vitamin D deficient, as defined by a 25-OH-D concentration <25 nmol/L (van der Meer, Karamali, & Boeke, 2006).

Maternal and Corresponding Fetal Vitamin D Levels: One aspect of vitamin D metabolism that has been substantiated by multiple studies is the strong relationship between maternal and fetal (cord blood) circulating 25(OH)D levels (Bouillon, Van Baelen, & DeMoor, 1977; Bouillon, Van Assche, Van Baelen, Heyns, & DeMoor, 1981; Hollis & Pittard, 1984; Markestad, Aksnes, Ulstein, & Aarskog, 1984). Our group demonstrated that vitamin D status at birth is closely related to that of the mother and is greatly influenced by race (Hollis & Pittard, 1984). The data revealed that the fetus at birth (cord blood) will contain approximately 60% of the maternal circulating levels of 25(OH)D. This relationship appears to be linear, even at pharmacological intakes of vitamin D (Greer, Hollis, & Napoli, 1984).

As far as the more polar metabolites of vitamin D, a similar (but lesser) relationship is observed between mother and fetus (Hollis & Pittard, 1984). Interestingly, there appears to be little, if any, relationship with respect to the parent vitamin, vitamin

D (Hollis & Pittard, 1984). This lack of placental transfer of the parent vitamin D from mother to fetus has also been observed in a porcine experimental animal model, adding further validation to what we have seen in humans (Goff, Horst, & Littledike, 1984). **Thus, in the human fetus, vitamin D metabolism in all likelihood begins with 25(OH)D.** As a result, the nutritional vitamin D status of the human fetus/neonate mirrors that of the mother (Hollis & Pittard, 1984); thus, if the mother is hypovitaminotic D, her fetus will experience depleted vitamin D exposure throughout gestation.

Health Implications of Vitamin D for the Pregnant Woman and Her Developing Fetus

As we discussed in **Section 8** regarding the health implications of vitamin D status, higher circulating 25(OH)D levels have been linked with improved glucose handling and beta-cell function (Chiu et al., 2004) and a growing list of long latency diseases that include cardiovascular disease (Zittermann, Schleithoff, & Koerfer, 2005; Giovannucci et al., 2006; Zittermann et al., 2006; Forman et al., 2007; Giovannucci et al., 2008), multiple sclerosis (Hayes, 2000; Munger et al., 2006; Kimball et al., 2007), rheumatoid arthritis (Merlino et al., 2004), systemic lupus erythematosus (Kamen et al., 2006), Type 1 and 2 diabetes (Merlino et al., 2004), and at least 15 types of cancers (Garland et al., 1989; Garland et al., 1990; Rao, 1990; Lefkowitz & Garland, 1994; Grant, 2002; Rao, 2002; Holick, 2004; Egan et al., 2008; Freedman et al., 2008).

While these studies describe strong correlation with vitamin D deficiency and a diverse group of long latency diseases, they do not provide proof of causality or a mechanism of action and often lead to what is referred to as "circular epidemiology" (Morgan et al., 2009). Two studies have begun to decipher the riddle of vitamin D's role in maintaining the innate immune system with profound implications (Liu et al., 2006; Martineau et al., 2007). Some of this data, as well as additional studies, have been summarized in two recent reviews regarding the optimization of circulating 25(OH)D levels to reduce the risk of long latency disease states (Hollis, 2005; Holick, 2007b).

As we discussed earlier, in an ideal world, total circulating 25(OH)D should mirror what is attained by those who live and work in a sun-rich environment; those individuals have circulating 25(OH)D levels of 54-90 ng/mL (Haddad & Chyu, 1971; Haddock et al., 1982; Matsuoka, Wortsman, Hanifan, et al. 1988), not shared by those who are sunlight deprived or covered from sunlight (Hollis et al., 2007). The debate about what constitutes frank deficiency, insufficiency, and sufficiency continues, but less vehemently than 5 years ago. Depending on what biomarker one chooses, there could be a different cut point for each category. Most, however, would agree that levels below 50 nmol/L (or 20 ng/mL) represent deficiency; whether that label extends to 70 or even 80 nmol/L is less clear.

A clinical scenario that occurs millions of times daily throughout the world is the following: A pregnant woman visits her obstetrician, primary health care provider, or nurse midwife who prescribes prenatal vitamins containing 400 IU (10 µg) vitamin D. Both the patient and physician assume that this supplement will fulfill all the nutritional requirements for the duration of the pregnancy; however, in the case of vitamin D, this approach does not come close to meeting the needs of the woman unless she has adequate sun exposure. The woman, especially if African-American, and her developing fetus are at high risk of remaining vitamin D-deficient during the entire pregnancy (Nesby-O'Dell et al., 2002). Even if the physician were to prescribe a 1,000 IU (40 µg)/day vitamin D supplement, the mother would likely remain vitamin D-deficient (Mallet et al., 1986; Datta et al., 2002). It is only with doses above 2,000 IU vitamin D/day that a pregnant woman becomes replete in vitamin D. In our two prospective, randomized control trials involving more than 510 women, 4000 IU vitamin D/day was the most efficacious and effective in safely achieving total circulating 25(OH)D levels above 30 ng/mL in pregnant women (Wagner, Johnson, et al. 2010a; Wagner, McNeil, et al. 2010; Wagner, Johnson, et al. 2010b). In our modern world where more than 93% of our time is spent indoors, this is what it takes to safely make a pregnant woman, and by default, her developing fetus replete in vitamin D for the vast majority. The final results of such studies will allow the medical community to decipher this information, but until then, it is the onus of the primary care provider to make recommendations for each pregnant woman that above all do no harm, and that we might add includes avoiding vitamin D deficiency.

11. Vitamin D Requirements During Lactation

By Carol L. Wagner, M.D., Sarah N. Taylor, M.D., and Bruce W. Hollis, Ph.D.

Vitamin D and the Breastfeeding Mother-Infant Dyad: Are They Mutually Exclusive?

Human milk is a bridge between *in utero* and *ex utero* life. There is a natural progression from placental nutrition during pregnancy to human milk provided after delivery (Wagner, Taylor, & Johnson, 2008). For this reason, it is not surprising that human milk is considered the ideal nutrition for the neonate and growing infant with one caveat—for many babies, it lacks sufficient concentrations of one essential vitamin and hormonal—vitamin D (Gartner et al., 2003). The premise that human milk has low levels of vitamin D was born out of the observation that breastfed infants are at risk for rickets unless they are exposed to adequate sunlight or are supplemented orally with sufficient amounts of vitamin D (Ala-Houhala, 1985; Sills, Skuza, Horlick, Schwartz, & Rapaport, 1994; Binet & Kooh, 1996; Daaboul, Sanderson, Kristensen, & Kitson, 1997; Pugliese, Blumberg, Hludzinski, & Kay, 1998; Kreiter et al., 2000; Mylott, Kump, Bolton, & Greenbaum, 2004; Weisburg et al., 2004). Darkly pigmented infants and younger children, in particular, are at risk for vitamin D deficiency due to maternal deficiency during pregnancy and lactation, leading to less vitamin D reserve at delivery and lower levels of vitamin D in the breastmilk (Cancela, LeBoulch, & Miravet, 1986).

Our recent understanding of human vitamin D requirements—based on functional indicators of vitamin D activity—demonstrates that most of us, particularly women in their childbearing years, subsist in a vitamin D insufficient state—at best (Nesby-O'Dell et al., 2002). Evidence of widespread deficiency during pregnancy was found in our two pregnancy cohorts in South Carolina, a place that is sunny and closer to the equator at latitude 32°N (Wagner, Johnson, et al., 2008). Even with maternal supplementation of recommended daily intake of 400 IU/day of vitamin D$_3$, human milk contains only 33-68 IU/L levels of serum concentration, far below the required 200-800 IU/day to prevent rickets (Hollis, 1983; Greer, Hollis, Cripps, & Tsang, 1984; Hollis & Wagner 2004b; Wagner et al., 2006).

The question of giving more than 400 IU vitamin D/day to a nursing mother was not considered a viable option for fear of creating vitamin D toxicity in that mother; the efficacy and safety of maternal vitamin D supplementation to achieve vitamin D-sufficient human milk is based upon the assumption that maternal vitamin D toxicity occurs at a vitamin D dose above 2,000 IU/day, the upper limit of safety set by the Institute of Medicine (Narang et al., 1984; Standing Committee Dietary Reference Intakes, 1997). If we cannot safely give higher amounts of vitamin D to mothers, if we cannot recommend sunlight exposure to mothers, then we must recommend supplementation to those infants and children at greatest risk for vitamin D deficiency. In the following sections, we review why these points of views have come about and what the controversies are.

Defining Infant Vitamin D Requirements

The first controversy to highlight is **HUGE**: what constitutes sufficiency in neonates, infants, and children? When we viewed vitamin D's role as exclusive to bone metabolism and the prevention of rickets, it was much easier, albeit wrong, to define vitamin D deficiency as that point at which rickets could be prevented (Weick, 1967). Deficiency then was defined as circulating 25(OH)D levels above 10-11 ng/mL (25-27.5 nmol/L). But science is not static and we have come to realize that there is more to vitamin D than rickets. So, let us repeat the question in the context of the 21st century—what constitutes sufficiency in neonates, infants, and children?

A daily dose of 400 IU vitamin D per day has a long record of reliably preventing infantile rickets, yet even for that established dose, the documentation of vitamin D adequacy is scant—most of the pertinent studies occurred before it was possible to measure vitamin D status accurately and consistently (Park, 1923; Hess, 1929; Park, 1940). In addition, with the ongoing, new developments in our understanding of the vitamin D requirements in adults, we are beginning to realize that vitamin D sufficiency cannot be defined simply as the absence of rickets or osteoporosis (Vieth et al., 2007). In evaluation of the long-term effect of infant vitamin D status, one retrospective cohort study demonstrated a significant association between vitamin D supplementation during infancy and bone mineral mass at specific skeletal sites in prepubertal girls (Zamora, Rizzoli, Belli, Slosman, & Bonjour, 1999). Another series of studies by Hypponen et al. (Hypponen et al., 2001; Hypponen, 2004; Hypponen et al., 2004) brought to light how vitamin D status during infancy may have far-reaching effects on outcomes other than bone health. In this now 30-year prospective cohort study of 10,821 infants born in Finland, there was an 80% decrease in the risk of diabetes mellitus Type I in infants who received at least 2,000 IU vitamin D per day in the first year of life (Hypponen et al., 2001; Hypponen et al., 2004). The findings from this large epidemiological study suggest that there was an early life effect either from vitamin D itself or something associated with vitamin D (where vitamin D is the indicator) that decreased the autoimmune-inflammatory processes that ultimately lead to Type 1-diabetes. Long before this association was made, there was evidence of vitamin D's role in immune function (Rook, 1986; Rook et al., 1986; Poulter, Rook, Steele, & Condez, 1987; Rook & Steele, 1987; Rook, Taverne, Leveton, & Steele, 1987; Rook, 1988; Bahr et al., 1989). It would take another twenty years to really sort out the mechanistic role that vitamin D plays via cathelicidin, whose product—LL37 is an antimicrobial peptide capable of killing bacteria (Liu et al., 2006). (Please refer to **Section 5** for a more detailed discussion of the topic.)

With current infant formula and vitamin D supplements providing 400 IU/day (Mead Johnson, 2004; Atkinson & Tsang, 2005) and recent recommendations for infants to receive 400 IU/day ("Vitamin D supplementation,"2007; Wagner & Greer, 2008), understanding the expected effect of 400 IU/day is essential. We have decades of experience with the 1 teaspoon per day of cod liver oil, but no laboratory parameters to validate our claim, other than "there were no reports of toxicity." We begin the process of presenting those clinical trials that were conducted with associated circulating 25(OH)D and other metabolites and have summarized those available trials in **Table 1**. Of note, in the study published by Pittard et al. in 1991, 80% of the subjects were African American. In addition, in that study, a second group of term infants received 800 IU/day vitamin D with resulting mean serum 25(OH)D of 35 ng/ml at 16 weeks.

Table 1. Studies Evaluating a Dose of 400 IU/Day Vitamin D in Early Infancy

Studies	Serum 25(OH)D with no vitamin D supplement	Serum 25(OH)D with 400 IU/day vitamin D	Length of Supplementation
Greer et al., 1982	12.9 ng/mL	32.7 ng/mL	6 months
Greer et al., 1989 (90)	23.5	37	6 months
Pittard et al., 1991	Not studied	26	16 weeks
Wagner et al., 2006	At one month: 13 ng/mL	43 ng/mL	12 weeks
Wagner et al., 2010	At one month: 16.0± 9.3 ng/mL (range 1.0-40.8; n=33)	At 4 months: 43.6 ± 14.1 (range 18.2-69.7) At 7 months: 42.5 ± 12.1 ng/mL (range 18.9-67.2)	16 weeks 24 weeks (6 months)

Adapted from Taylor, Wagner, & Hollis., 2008, p. 695. Reproduced with permission from American Society for Nutrition.

In a related study of vitamin D supplementation in infancy, Zeghoud et al. (1997) provided 500 and 1,000 vitamin D IU/day above that was received with 426 IU vitamin D/L formula. The investigators classified the infants into three groups based on vitamin D and intact parathyroid hormone (iPTH) status at birth and evaluated the infants at 1 and 3 months. They reported that infants with serum 25(OH)D ≤ 12 ng/mL and iPTH > 60 ng/L (vitamin D deficient) had a mean serum 25(OH)D of 18.2 ng/mL at 1 month and 22.4 ng/mL at 3 months when receiving 500 IU vitamin D/day plus formula. For the vitamin D deficient infants who received 1,000 IU vitamin D/day plus formula, serum 25(OH)D status was 21.2 ng/ml at 1 month. In the group of infants who demonstrated serum 25(OH)D ≤ 12 ng/ml at birth, but had normal iPTH (< 60 ng/L) and received 1000 IU vitamin D/day plus formula, the serum 25(OH)D rose to 23.9 ng/ml by 1 month. In the group of infants with serum 25(OH)D > 12 ng/ml at birth who received 1,000 IU/day vitamin D plus formula, serum 25(OH)D was 23.7 ng/ml at 1 month. In this study, serum calcium, iPTH, alkaline phosphatase activity, and phosphate were monitored with no evidence of vitamin D toxicity.

Although the number of studies is few, collectively these studies demonstrate that 400 - 1426 IU vitamin D/day supplementation can be given to infants without toxicity and with vitamin D status above the range associated with infantile rickets. We remain rather in the dark about what amount of supplementation will achieve optimal vitamin D status in infants and young children within a certain margin of safety. Such answers will only come from careful and methodical clinical studies.

History Repeats Itself: Breastfeeding's Effect on Infant Vitamin D Status and Its Relationship to Nutritional Rickets

Thirty-five years ago, the incidence of nutritional rickets was thought to be disappearing (Harrison, 1996). Since then, however, there have been many reports, beginning in the 1980s, that indicate otherwise (Bachrach, Fisher, & Parks, 1979; Elidrissy, Sedrani, & Lawson, 1984; Taha, Dost, & Sedrani, 1984; Sills et al., 1994; Eugster, Sane, & Brown, 1996; Kreiter et al., 2000; Welch, Bergstrom, & Tsang, 2000; Kreiter, 2001; Scanlon, 2001; Tomashek et al., 2001; Dawodu, Agarwal, Hossain, Kochiyil, & Zayed, 2003; NIH, 2003; Weisburg et al., 2004; Alouf & Grigalonis, 2005; Balasubramanian, Shivbalan, & Kumar, 2006; Dawodu & Tsang, 2007; Dawodu & Wagner, 2007; Saadi et al., 2007; Ward, Gaboury, Ladhani, & Zlotkin, 2007). The majority of the cases reported have involved darkly pigmented infants who were exclusively breastfed. Hollis et al. previously showed that vitamin D status at birth is closely related to that of the mother and is related to race (Hollis & Pittard, 1984). These data from more than two decades ago clearly demonstrated that urban African American women and their infants have circulating 25(OH)D levels well below what constitutes vitamin D sufficiency as it is defined today (Hollis, 2005). Recent studies confirm the widespread deficiency that is present in women during their childbearing years (Nesby-O'Dell et al., 2002), during pregnancy (Wagner, Johnson, et al. 2008; Johnson et al., 2010 in press), and in their newborn infants at delivery (Basile, Taylor, Quinones, Wagner, & Hollis, 2007). The implications of that deficiency are no longer limited to rickets, but extend to every organ system through vitamin D's effect on the innate immune system (Liu et al., 2006).

Vitamin D Content of Human Milk and Factors Affecting Content

From antiquity to modern times, human milk was viewed as an adequate source of antirachitic activity for the growing infant, with rickets typically appearing after a mother weaned her infant from the breast. Even before the true identify of vitamin D was discovered, McCollum et al. (1922) and Park (1923) stated that rickets was due to the deprivation of sunlight and a dietary factor X. They observed that factor X was found in "good breastmilk" and cod liver oil, and that although rickets did develop in breastfed children, it was rarely as severe as in artificially fed infants. As was discussed in Section 4, early attempts to quantify the antirachitic potential (or anti-rickets effect, which is the sum total of all vitamin D and its metabolites) of human milk were crude and yielded little information (Drummond et al., 1939; Harris & Bunket, 1939; Polskin, Kramer, & Sobel, 1945). For a time, it was believed that vitamin D sulfate was responsible for the antirachitic activity in human milk (Sahshi, Suzuki, Higaki, & Asano, 1967; Lakdawala & Widdowson, 1977); however, this was shown not to be the case (Hollis, Roos, Drapper, & Lambert, 1981a). The 1980s were a time of technological advances that allowed the analysis of technically challenging fluids with high lipid content, such as human milk. It was during this time that the concentrations of vitamin D and its metabolites could be measured.

Concurrent with the increasing reports of rickets in breastfed infants in the 1980s, the antirachitic activity of human milk from mothers receiving 400 IU vitamin D/ day was found to be low, at 20-70 IU/L (Hollis, Roos, & Lambert, 1981; Reeve, Chesney, & Deluca, 1982; Hollis, 1983), with the conclusion made that human milk had minimally sufficient levels of vitamin D and its metabolites. This content was first reliably measured in the early 1980's by ligand binding analysis (Hollis, Roos, Drapper, et al. 1981,a,b; Hollis, Roos, & Lambert, 1981). As mentioned earlier, previous assays that were adequate for serum analysis did not possess the sensitivity required to evaluate the vitamin D activity in human milk (Drummond et al., 1939; Harris & Bunket, 1939; Polskin et al., 1945).

The difficulty in measuring vitamin D or antirachitic activity in human milk compared to serum is that native milk contains only a small percentage of the circulating sterols that are present in serum, and milk contains an enormous amount of lipid compared to blood. If present, this lipid can interfere with the ligand binding assays for vitamin D and give falsely elevated results. Therefore, the functional assays refined by Dr. Hollis involved alkalinization of the milk for removal of lipids, followed by exhaustive high performance liquid chromatography

(HPLC) to separate and purify these antirachitic sterols, and then ligand binding assays to determine the content of vitamin D_3, vitamin D_2, and their metabolites (Hollis, Roos, Drapper, et al. 1981a,b; Hollis, Roos, & Lambert, 1982; Hollis, 1986; Hollis, Pittard, & Reinhardt, 1986).

In an article by Hollis et al. published in 1986, the relationship between circulating vitamin D_2, D_3, 25(OH)D_2 and 25(OH)D_3, and corresponding milk levels in 51 lactating mothers was described (Hollis et al., 1986). The relationship between circulating blood and milk concentrations of various vitamin D sterols were examined by regression analysis. The two essential forms of vitamin D in human milk, vitamin D and 25(OH)D, have specific functions based on their metabolism and their interrelation with vitamin D binding protein, DBP.

As was discussed in **Section 7**, DBP is an alpha globulin that binds vitamin D metabolites with varying affinities (Hollis & Horst, 2007; Zella, Shevde, Hollis, Cooke, & Pike, 2008). DBP's highest association is with 25(OH)D, which promotes a consistent circulating concentration of 25(OH)D, with minimal day-to-day variation due to UVB exposure or vitamin D intake (Haddad & Hahn, 1973; Haddad & Stamp, 1974; Hollis et al., 1986). On the other hand, the parent compound, vitamin D, can demonstrate great variability in circulating concentration with UVB exposure or fluctuation in vitamin D intake. Human milk is ideally created to benefit from the properties of both compounds. The concentration of 25(OH)D in human milk, which represents approximately 1% of the maternal circulating 25(OH)D provides a steady supply of antirachitic activity that is resistant to daily changes in vitamin D supply. In contrast, 20-30% of maternal circulating vitamin D is expressed in human milk. This expression allows maternal variation in vitamin D metabolite due to UVB exposure or fluctuations in intake to be transferred into the milk (Greer, Hollis, Cripps, et al. 1984; Specker, Tsang, & Hollis, 1985; Hollis et al., 1986).

There is a significant correlation seen in regression analyses between vitamin D_2 in maternal serum and human milk. Similar significant relationships have been found between plasma and milk concentrations of vitamin D_3, 25(OH)D_2, and 25(OH)D_3. In contrast, the plasma D-binding protein (DBP) levels are not related in these fluids. The parent vitamins gained access into the milk much more readily than their 25-hydroxylated metabolites: vitamin D in milk is approximately 20% of the plasma concentration, whereas 25(OH)D in milk is approximately 0.5-1.0% of that in plasma. Prior studies suggest that 25(OH)D is the most stable antirachitic compound, whereas vitamin D is the compound that provides the greatest potential for "adjustment" of antirachitic activity in milk (Hollis, 1983; Greer, Hollis, Cripps, et al. 1984; Greer, Hollis, & Napoli, 1984; Hollis et al., 1986).

We know today that the transfer of the antirachitic sterols from the circulation to milk is most likely a function of their ability to associate with the plasma DBP. As we discussed in **Section 5**, the DBP functions as a "sink" for vitamin D and its metabolites, and the vast majority of these antirachitic sterols are bound by this globulin in the circulation (Haddad & Stamp, 1974). The antirachitic sterols can only enter a cell by diffusion once they are dissociated from their carrier protein (DBP). This is referred to as the "free concentration" of the sterol and follows the law of mass action[12] (Bikle et al., 1986). The free concentration of the sterol is determined by two factors: 1) the sterol's affinity to bind to the DBP, and 2) the concentration of the DBP in the circulation.

The higher the binding affinity of the sterol towards the DBP, the lower the free concentration of the sterol and the less sterol available for cell membrane translocation, or in other words, less transfer into the milk. This translocation of vitamin D from blood to milk probably occurs through a lipoprotein-containing particle, much like that of cholesterol (Monks et al., 2001). From previous work, we know that the association constant for the antirachitic sterols with the DBP is far greater for 25(OH)D than vitamin D (Hollis, 1984). Thus, this model predicts what has been observed: the circulating parent vitamin D gains access to milk at a much greater rate than does the 25-hydroxylated metabolite. Given that, which form of the vitamin is most important in determining the antirachitic properties of milk? The data suggest that the role of 25(OH)D is to supply a relatively stable amount of antirachitic activity into milk, which appears to be dictated by two factors:

---

[12] The law of mass action is a statement about kinetics. The law states that the rate of an elementary reaction (a reaction that proceeds through only one transition state, that is one mechanistic step) is proportional to the product of the concentrations of the participating molecules, in this case 25(OH)D and vitamin D.

(1) Circulating levels of 25(OH)D are stable for relatively long periods of time (t½ ~3 wks), and therefore, are not influenced greatly by day-to-day sun exposure or dietary changes.

(2) The transfer of 25(OH)D from circulation to milk is greatly limited by the circulating DBP that binds 25(OH)D with high affinity and thus limits its free concentration and translocation across the mammary complex into the milk.

These data have a practical implication: The vitamin D content of human milk is directly related to the lactating mother's vitamin D status. *Vitamin D status—in this case—refers to both circulating vitamin D and 25(OH)D.* In lactating mothers taking 400 IU/day vitamin D, we found human milk to contain 33-68 IU/L antirachitic activity (Hollis et al., 1986; Wagner et al., 2006). This was verified by our recent supplementation study of women at baseline taking 400 IU/day vitamin D (n=35), whose milk had a mean antirachitic activity of 37.9±10.7 IU/L (Hollis & Wagner 2004b). These calculations were based on various conversion factors for the biological activity of 25(OH)D.[13] Both the parent vitamin and the 25-hydroxylated form contribute significantly to the antirachitic properties of human milk.

Effect of Sunlight Exposure on Milk's Vitamin D Content

With knowledge that human milk concentrations of vitamin D and 25(OH)D correspond to the maternal circulating levels of these compounds, studies have also demonstrated that human milk vitamin D activity relies completely on maternal vitamin D status achieved either by UV exposure or oral supplementation (Greer, Hollis, Cripps, et al. 1984; Greer, Hollis, & Napoli, 1984; Specker, Valanis, Hertzberg, Edwards, & Tsang, 1985; Cancela et al., 1986). Trying to sort out the effect of each source of vitamin D, the question of sunlight's effect on vitamin D content in human milk then becomes important. It was addressed by Greer et al. in their study of lactating women (Greer, Hollis, Cripps, et al., 1984).

---

[13] All biological assays are based on the parent vitamin containing 1 IU activity (25 ng) (Tanaka et al., 1973), with some disagreement, however, with regard to the biological activity of 25(OH)D with 1 IU equaling between 5 and 18 ng depending on the biological assay (Tanaka et al., 1973; Reeve et al., 1982).

Following total body UVB exposure of lactating women equal to 30 minutes of sunshine at midday on a clear summer day at temperate latitudes, Greer et al. found increasing vitamin D_3 concentrations in the circulation and milk peaked within 48 hrs, followed by a rapid decline in both fluids due to the relatively short $t_{1/2}$ of the parent vitamin in the circulation (Greer, Hollis, Cripps, et al., 1984). Of note, due to the appearance of vitamin D_3 following simulated sunlight, antirachitic activity in mother's milk increased several fold. Not unexpected based on pharmacokinetic studies, in these same subjects, circulating $25(OH)D_3$ concentrations also increased from 13.9 to 20.5 ng/mL and remained significantly elevated for at least 14 days, but there was no significant change in the milk 25(OH)D concentrations. This study highlights the role of the parent compound, vitamin D, in human milk antirachitic activity and the requirement of consistent vitamin D dosing that reflects the relatively short half-life of this compound. Again, an important message from this study is the rapid decline in circulating and milk vitamin D_3 concentrations following a single phototherapy session due to the short parent vitamin $t_{1/2}$ in the circulation, and that for the lactating woman, consistent delivery of vitamin D— either through prudent sunlight exposure or oral vitamin D supplementation— will provide optimal vitamin D for her recipient breastfeeding infant.

Antirachitic Activity of Human Milk

From the prior discussions in this book, it is clear that the antirachitic content of human milk is quite variable and is affected by season, sunlight or ultraviolet exposure, maternal vitamin D intake, use of protective clothing or sunscreen, and race. Yet, they all have one thing in common: these factors dictate the sum total vitamin D status of the mother who is producing the milk, and she in turn dictates the vitamin D status of her milk. This premise is supported by the meticulous studies of Cancela et al. (1986), who reported that circulating 25(OH)D levels in breastfed infants are directly related to the vitamin D content of mother's milk. This was also shown by Hollis and colleagues (Hollis et al., 1986; Hollis & Wagner 2004b; Wagner et al., 2006).

Greer and Marshall (1989) reported that exclusively breastfed Caucasian infants who nursed during the winter in a northern climate maintained a "minimally normal" vitamin D status for a period of 6 months. During the study, as would be expected by the seasonal variation that is witnessed at higher latitudes, such as Ohio, circulating 25(OH)D levels in the breastfeeding infants from the Greer study actually declined as winter progressed. This decline occurred in spite of a maternal vitamin D intake of approximately 700 IU/day (Greer & Marshall, 1989).

Specker et al. (Specker, Tsang, et al., 1985) determined that the antirachitic content of human milk was lower in African American mothers than in Caucasian mothers. This difference was attributed to variation in dietary intake of vitamin D and UV exposure. As more research was done in the field of vitamin D, it became more apparent that degree of pigmentation had much effect on overall vitamin D status of the mother and thus of the vitamin D in her milk and that transferred to her breastfeeding infant via her milk (Hollis & Wagner, 2004a; Hollis & Wagner, 2004b; Wagner et al., 2006).

How much vitamin D is actually delivered to the milk from the mother is an important question. It is answered in part by a case report of a woman with a history of hypoparathyroidism before the days of parathyroid hormone (PTH) replacement. In this case, the woman became pregnant and was maintained on 100,000 IU/day vitamin D_2 for the maintenance of plasma calcium (Greer, Hollis, & Napoli, 1984). She subsequently delivered a normal child at term and then breastfed her infant for 2 weeks. At that point, the mother's milk contained approximately 7,600 IU of antirachitic activity (**Table 2**)!

Table 2. Concentration of Vitamin D_2, D_3, 25(OH)D_2 and 25(OH)D_3 in Maternal And Neonatal Cord Serum and Mother's Milk from a Mother Receiving 100,000 IU/day Vitamin D_2

Serum Type	Vitamin D_2 (ng/mL)	Vitamin D_3 (ng/mL)	25(OH)D_2 (ng/mL)	25(OH)D_3 (ng/mL)	IU/L*
Maternal [At delivery]	551	<1	545	4.9	
Cord	46	<1	251	2.0	
Breastmilk [14 days]	155	<1	7.3	<0.01	7,660

*Estimated using conversion factors 25 ng vitamin D = 1 IU and 5 ng 25(OH)D = 1 IU

From Taylor, Wagner, & Hollis, 2008. Reprinted with permission from American Society for Nutrition.

Of this activity, the parent vitamin (vitamin D) accounted for approximately 81%, with 25(OH)D metabolite accounting for 19%. It is interesting to note that the circulating levels of vitamin D and 25(OH)D were almost identical in the mother, yet a much higher percentage of the parent compound passed into the milk. This mother's milk contained vitamin D at 30% of her circulating concentration of vitamin D and 25(OH)D at 1% of her circulating concentration of 25(OH)D. This case report and results from recent clinical trials show that, for human milk to achieve vitamin D sufficient status in the recipient infant, the parent compound vitamin D is the responsible form (Hollis & Wagner, 2004b).

High-Dose Maternal Supplementation

While the case of the woman with hypoparathyroidism above is extreme, its relevance to normal subjects must be underscored. This case report leads to the next question: if vitamin D supplementation in this woman did effectively increase her milk antirachitic activity, could other women be supplemented with vitamin D to achieve the same effect in their breastmilk and thus in their breastfeeding infants?

Unfortunately, the answer to that question is not so easy. Scientific data pertaining to vitamin D supplementation during lactation in the human subject is extremely scarce. An arbitrary AI had been set at 400 IU/day for the lactating mother, and this AI continues to present (Institute of Medicine, 1990b). The few studies that have been published on the effect of maternal vitamin D supplementation on the 25(OH)D status of infant's receiving complete human milk nutrition have shown an evolution in thinking. The early studies bounded by the concern that maternal intakes above 2000 IU/day had a high likelihood of toxicity not surprisingly found no significant improvement with 500-1000 IU/day vitamin D$_2$ intake (Rothberg, Pettifor, Cohen, Sonnendecker, & Ross, 1982; Ala-Houhala, 1985; Ala-Houhala, Koskinen, Terho, Koivula, & Visakorpi, 1986; Takeuchi et al., 1989; Tomashek et al., 2001).

One group of investigators in Finland headed by Ala-Houhala published a series of papers (1985-1988) comparing maternal vitamin D$_3$ intakes of 1,000 and 2,000 IU/day with infant intake of 400 IU/day (Ala-Houhala, 1985; Ala-Houhala et al., 1986; Ala-Houhala, Koskinen, Parviainen & Visakorpi, 1988). The rise in circulating 25(OH)D levels in the infants during this period of supplementation was 16 and 23 ng/mL for the maternal 1,000 and 2,000 IU dose groups, respectively. This result compared favorably to the infants receiving 400 IU/day whose serum 25(OH)D increased from a mean of 8.5 ng/mL at birth to a mean above 30 ng/ml at 15 postnatal weeks. Their mothers, who received no supplementation, had no change in their mean serum 25(OH)D level of 11 ng/mL. For the infants who received no direct supplementation of vitamin D and whose mothers received 1000 IU/day vitamin D_3, serum 25(OH)D rose over 15 weeks from a mean of 8.5 ng/ml to 15 ng/ml, but despite this increase, this concentration was significantly lower than that observed for both the infants whose mothers received 2000 IU/day and the infants who directly received 400 IU/day. Specifically, maternal supplementation with 2,000 IU/day vitamin D_3 for 15 weeks increased maternal serum 25(OH)D from a mean of 11 ng/mL to close to 40 ng/mL. In the infants being exclusively breastfed during this time with maternal milk as their only source with no additional vitamin D intake, the serum 25(OH)D increased from a mean of 8.5 ng/mL at birth to a mean nearing 30 ng/mL. When comparing foremilk to hindmilk, there was greater antirachitic activity in the hindmilk, due to the higher fat content (Ala-Houhala et al., 1988). In these studies, it was clear that maternal supplementation with 2000 IU/day was superior to the 400 or 1000 IU/day regimen. In their conclusions, however, the authors added the following disclaimer:

> *A sufficient supply of vitamin D to the breastfed infant is achieved only by increasing the maternal supplementation up to 2,000 IU/day. As such, (this) dose is far higher than the daily dietary allowance recommended for lactating mothers (and therefore,) its safety over prolonged periods is not known and should be examined (p. 1163).*

These results were lost in the catacombs of libraries and electronic files for two decades, partly due to the concern of toxicity in prescribing the "tolerable upper intake limit" of 2,000 IU/day to lactating women (Ala-Houhala, 1985; Ala-Houhala et al., 1986; Institute of Medicine, 1990a; Institute of Medicine, 1990b; Hollis & Wagner, 2004a), and the ambiguity of what circulating 25(OH)D level actually connotes vitamin D sufficiency in mothers and infants (Hollis, 2005; Hollis et al., 2007). As we saw from the careful work of Ala-Houhala et al. (Ala-

Houhala, 1985; Ala-Houhala et al., 1986; Ala-Houhala et al., 1988), maternal supplementation with 1000 IU vitamin D_3 per day did increase serum 25(OH) D concentration in infants to a level considered sufficient to avoid rickets (15 ng/ mL), but not even this concentration of maternal supplementation was adopted.

With a change in our perspective about the role of vitamin D within our bodies, the paradigm of what constitutes sufficiency and toxicity is changing. Studies continue to demonstrate that even 2,000 IU vitamin D/day does not represent adequate supplementation for certain adults (Vieth, Chan, et al., 2001; Vieth, Cole, et al., 2001; Hollis, 2005; Whiting & Calvo, 2005; "Vitamin D supplementation,"2007; Vieth et al., 2007; Ward et al., 2007). With this improved understanding of human vitamin D needs, reexamination of the question—can human milk attain adequate vitamin D status—has occurred.

Following the landmark studies of Vieth et al. (Vieth, 1999; Vieth, Chan, et al., 2001), it was possible to conduct high-dose vitamin D supplementation trials in lactating women. We conducted the first pilot trial starting in February 2001 in exclusively or fully lactating mothers randomized to receive either 2,000 or 4,000 IU vitamin D_2/day for 3 months (Hollis & Wagner, 2004). Blood, urine and milk samples were obtained monthly from the mothers. Infant blood was collected at months 1 and 4 of Study 1. Serum from each mother was monitored for total calcium, phosphorus, vitamins D_2, D_3, 25(OH)D_2, and 25(OH)D_3. Infant serum was monitored for vitamins D_2, D_3, 25(OH)D_2, and 25(OH)D_3, calcium, and phosphorus. Mother's urine was monitored for calcium/creatinine ratio as a first line measure of potential vitamin D toxicity[14] and milk was assessed for vitamin D antirachitic activity by measuring vitamin D_2, D_3, 25(OH)D_2, and 25(OH) D_3. Vitamin D_2 was used for maternal dosing as a specific tracking agent since the contribution of D_2 is very small, as foods are fortified with vitamin D_3 and not D_2. By using vitamin D_2 in this study which was measured at each visit, we precisely defined the rise and/or transfer of vitamin D compounds in/from the mother to her infant without confounding factors, such as extra dietary intake (in the form

[14] Urinary calcium/creatinine ratio increases during hypervitaminosis D as the body attempts to normalize the serum calcium level by "dumping" extra calcium in the urine. This is the first sign of excess vitamin D. If unchecked, the serum calcium level will begin to rise, and hypercalcemia becomes the second and more dangerous sign of hypervitaminosis D or vitamin D toxicity. The calcium then begins to fall out of solution and calcifications in every organ system, but especially in bone, intestine and kidneys are appreciated.

of vitamin D_3) and sun exposure (which leads to vitamin D_3 in humans). This is shown in **Figures 3-8**.

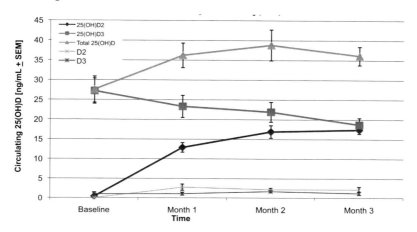

Figure 3. Circulating vitamin D concentrations (mean ± SEM) over time in lactating mothers receiving 1,600 IU/day vitamin D_2 and 400 IU/day vitamin D_3 (n=9).

From Hollis & Wagner, 2004b. Figure used with permission from American Society for Nutrition.

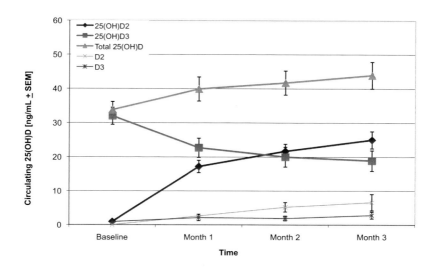

Figure 4. Circulating vitamin D concentrations (mean ± SEM) over time in lactating mothers receiving 3,600 IU/day vitamin D_2 and 400 IU/day vitamin D_3 (n=9).

From Hollis & Wagner, 2004b. Figure used with permission from American Society for Nutrition.

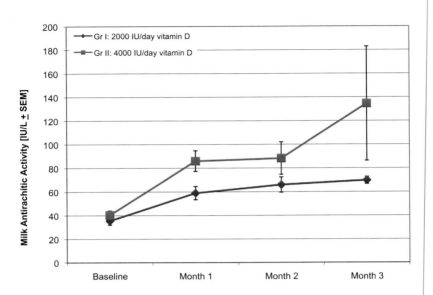

Figure 5. Whole milk samples were assessed for vitamin D antirachitic activity by measuring vitamin D_2, D_3, 25(OH)D_2 and 25(OH)D_3 concentrations in the milk, and converted into biological activity using reference data from biological activity assays. The mean (± SEM) milk antirachitic activity over time in lactating mothers receiving 2,000 or 4,000 IU/day vitamin D (n=18) is shown in this figure.

From Hollis & Wagner, 2004b. Figure used with permission from American Society for Nutrition.

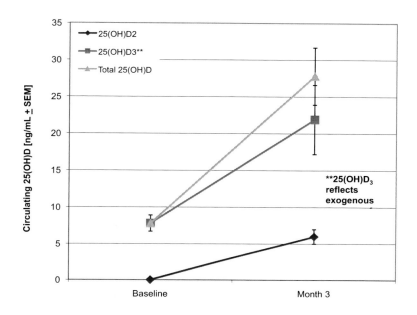

Figure 6. Circulating 25(OH)D concentrations (mean ± SEM) over time in nursing infants of mothers receiving 1,600 IU/day vitamin D_2 and 400 IU/day vitamin D_3 (n=9).

From Hollis & Wagner, 2004b. Figure used with permission from American Society for Nutrition.

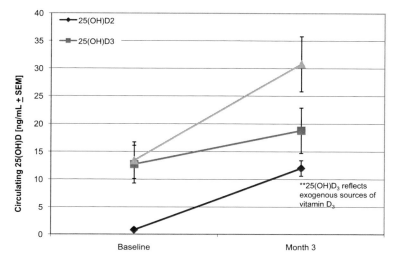

Figure 7. Circulating 25(OH)D concentrations (mean ± SEM) over time in nursing infants of mothers receiving 3,600 IU/day vitamin D_2 and 400 IU/day vitamin D_3 (n=8).

From Hollis & Wagner, 2004b. Figure used with permission from American Society for Nutrition.

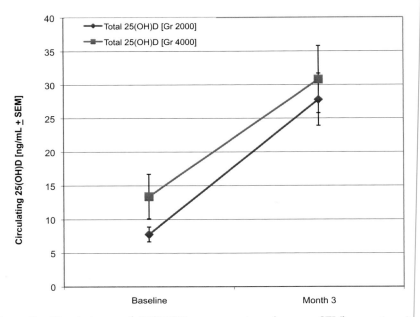

Figure 8. Circulating total 25(OH)D concentrations (mean ± SEM) over time in nursing infants of mothers receiving either 2,000 or 4,000 IU total vitamin D/day.

From Hollis & Wagner, 2004b. Figure used with permission from American Society for Nutrition.

In this study, we found that while this daily supplementation regimen in lactating mothers did raise the antirachitic activity of their breastmilk, with significantly greater effect in the 4,000 IU group; even in the 4000 IU group higher-dose group, milk antirachitic activity did not rise consistently above 200 IU/L (Hollis & Wagner, 2004b). The levels were less than predicted by pharmacokinetics, which may be explained by the observation that in some circumstances vitamin D_2 appears inferior to vitamin D_3 at maintaining circulating 25(OH)D levels in humans (Armas, Hollis, & Heaney, 2004).

Given the pharmacokinetics and transfer rates into milk, we theorized that 6,400 IU vitamin D/day would be the ideal supplementation regimen. To test this hypothesis, we conducted a subsequent pilot study of high-dose maternal supplementation with 6,400 IU vitamin D_3/day (Wagner et al., 2006). In our second pilot study, fully lactating women (n=19) were enrolled at 1-month postpartum into a randomized-control pilot trial. Each mother received one of two treatments for a 6-month study period: 0 or 6,000 IU vitamin D_3 plus a prenatal vitamin containing 400 IU vitamin D_3. The infants of mothers assigned to the control group received 300 IU vitamin D_3/day; those infants of mothers in the high dose group received 0 IU (placebo). Maternal serum and milk vitamin D and 25(OH)D were measured at baseline, then monthly; infant serum vitamin D and 25(OH)D were measured at baseline, and at months 4 and 7. Urinary calcium/creatinine ratios were measured monthly in both mothers and infants. Dietary and breastfeeding history and outdoor activity questionnaires were completed at each visit. In both pilot studies, maternal supplementation with high-dose vitamin D (2000, 4000, or 6400 IU vitamin D/day) safely resulted in increases in maternal circulating 25(OH)D concentrations and in milk anti-rachitic activity (Hollis & Wagner, 2004b; Wagner et al., 2006); however, only the 6400 IU/day regimen consistently increased maternal 25(OH)D and vitamin D levels in milk to achieve adequate levels in the recipient infant.

As shown in **Figures 9-11**, high-dose (6,400 IU/day) vitamin D_3 safely and significantly increased maternal circulating 25(OH)D and vitamin D from baseline compared to controls ($p<0.0028$ and 0.0043, respectively). Not surprisingly, mean milk antirachitic activity of mothers receiving 400 IU vit D/day decreased to a nadir of 45.6 at visit 4 and varied little during the study period (45.6-78.6 IU/L), while the mean activity in the 6,400 IU/day group increased from 82 to 873 IU/L ($p<0.0003$; see **Figure 12**).

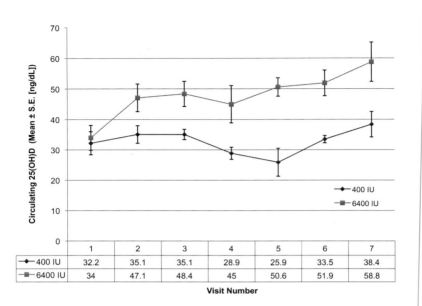

Figure 9. Maternal 25(OH)D Status: 400 IU vs. 6,400 IU Vitamin D₃/day Supplementation Regimen

From Wagner et al., 2006. Used with permission from Mary Ann Leibert, Inc.

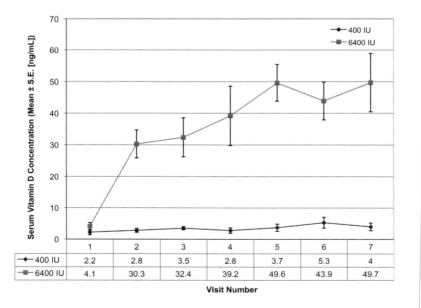

Figure 10. Maternal Serum Vitamin D Status: 400 IU vs. 6,400 IU Vitamin D₃/day Supplementation Regimen

From Wagner et al., 2006. Used with permission from Mary Ann Leibert, Inc.

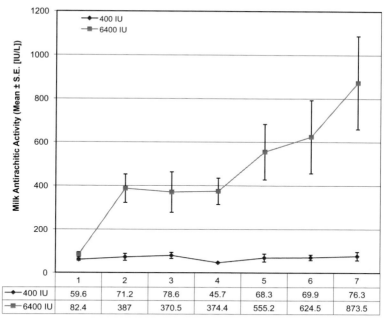

	1	2	3	4	5	6	7
400 IU	59.6	71.2	78.6	45.7	68.3	69.9	76.3
6400 IU	82.4	387	370.5	374.4	555.2	624.5	873.5

Visit Number

Figure 11. Milk Antirachitic Activity as a Function of Maternal Vitamin D$_3$ Dose: 400 vs. 6,400 IU/day

From Wagner et al., 2006. Used with permission from Mary Ann Leibert, Inc.

As shown in **Figure 12**, most significantly, there were no differences in circulating 25(OH)D levels of infants supplemented with oral vitamin D vs. infants whose only source of vitamin D was breastmilk. Infant levels achieved exclusively through maternal supplementation were equivalent to levels in infants who received oral vitamin D supplementation. Thus, a maternal intake of 6,400 IU vitamin D/day elevated circulating 25(OH)D in both mother and nursing infant, which resulted in a dramatic rise in infant circulating 25(OH) levels that mirrored levels of infants in that study receiving 300 IU vitamin D$_3$/day directly in drops. What is important to note is that this was achieved without toxicity to the mother.

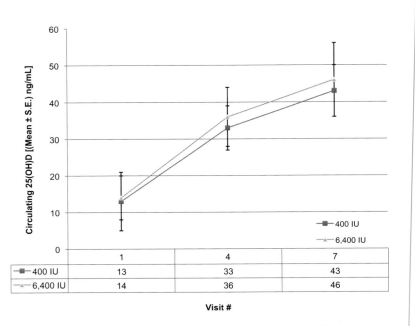

Figure 12. Infant Circulating 25(OH)D as a Function of Maternal Supplementation (400 vs. 6,400 IU vitamin D$_3$/day) and Infant Supplementation (300 vs. 0 IU vitamin D$_3$/day)

From Wagner et al., 2006. Used with permission from Mary Ann Leibert, Inc.

In our minds, the findings from this high-dose supplementation study reconfirm what is known about vitamin D pharmacokinetics and transfer into milk, and it strongly supports the premise that human milk is a mirror of maternal vitamin D status. And as we have said from the beginning, if mother is deficient in vitamin D, her milk will be deficient in vitamin D, and very logically, her infant will be deficient in vitamin D. Further, it was not surprising to find that in mothers with limited sun exposure, an intake of 400 IU/day vitamin D$_3$ did not sustain circulating maternal 25(OH)D levels, and thus, supplied only extremely limited amounts of vitamin D to the nursing infant via breastmilk. The mothers receiving only 400 IU/day exhibited a substantial decline in circulating 25(OH)D over a 3-month period during the winter months that placed them in a hypovitaminotic D state (Hollis, 2005). As a function of seasonality, these mothers' circulating 25(OH)D levels ultimately recovered later in the study due to increased UV exposure.

Another important point to mention from this second pilot study is the need for daily supplementation of vitamin D in lactating women. We made an interesting observation in one of our subjects ingesting 6,400 IU/day. Four days prior to visit 4 (3 months), this mother acquired an intestinal virus and was unable to take her supplement for 3 days prior to the scheduled visit. There was a rapid effect of the missed doses that was associated with a rapid decline of circulating vitamin D$_3$ and the resulting drop in milk antirachitic activity. This supports the premise that vitamin D$_3$ requires ingestion on a daily basis by the lactating mother to maintain her milk activity at maximum levels.

The two pilot studies led to our ongoing, two-site (Medical University of South Carolina and University of Rochester) NIH-sponsored vitamin D supplementation trial in lactating women and their infants (www.clinicaltrials.gov #NCT00412074) to further test the effectiveness and safety of these preliminary findings. While we remain blinded to treatment, this study is more than half completed, with no ill effects thus far seen with high-dose maternal vitamin D supplementation. As was predicted by the pharmacokinetics of vitamin D and prior studies by Ala-Houhala et al. (Ala-Houhala, 1985; Ala-Houhala et al., 1986; Ala-Houhala et al., 1988), transfer of vitamin D and its metabolites into breastmilk, and the subsequent transfer of antirachitic activity to the infant, the 2,000 IU arm of the study was stopped by our study's Data and Safety Monitoring Committee, as 50% of the infants in this arm required open-label vitamin D at 4 months compared with 5-6% in the other treatment arms (mother and infant on 400 IU vs. mother on 6,400 IU and infant on placebo drops).

At the very least, it is clear that the vitamin D content of human milk can be influenced by maternal diet and/or UV exposure. If a lactating mother has limited exposure, has darker pigmentation, and/or limited vitamin D intake (such as occurs with the current 400 IU/day AI and even up to 2,000 IU/day), the vitamin D content of her milk will be low. Given the rates of vitamin D deficiency and insufficiency in the United States today, particularly in women in their childbearing years, it is not surprising, then, that the milk antirachitic activity that is reliably measured is 20-70 IU/L. This activity in milk confirms what we have known for some time—that the mothers themselves are deficient and; therefore, there is not enough vitamin D to be passed to the recipient breastfeeding infant. While we have reviewed this subject previously in detail (Hollis, 2005), it is clear that larger, more detailed studies are required to confirm our findings and to determine the vitamin D requirement of the lactating mother.

How Can the Circulating Level of Maternal Vitamin D Be Kept Elevated for Extended Periods?

Very limited data exist on this point because frankly there was little attention in the past given to determining what sustained levels of vitamin D were. Rather, all of the attention was/is focused on 25(OH)D. *However, for a lactating mother, it is essential that sustained circulating vitamin D be maintained.* Again, sustained circulating vitamin D in the mother will result in a substantial increase in the vitamin D content of her milk. As we have just discussed, we estimate from our latest preliminary data that daily maternal intakes of 6,400 IU/day of vitamin D will result in raising the antirachitic activity of their milk to 500-800 IU/liter (Wagner et al., 2006). This level of antirachitic activity in human milk will likely be sufficient for the nursing infant to maintain adequate circulating levels of 25(OH) D. We are testing this hypothesis in an ongoing, two-site study in Charleston, South Carolina (latitude 32°N), and Rochester, New York (latitude 42°N). In the meantime, while we are waiting to find out both safety and effectiveness of high dose vitamin D supplementation in the lactating mother, what should one do? There are only two options—sunlight exposure with all its inherent risks and oral vitamin D supplementation in the infant and young child. Before we discuss how to make an infant and young child replete, we must discuss what vitamin D deficiency is and try to quantify the real risk of vitamin D deficiency in this age group.

Risk of Vitamin D Deficiency in Children

In the United Arab Emirates where the vast majority of women wear burkas, rates of rickets requiring hospitalization are high: 38 cases of infantile vitamin-D-deficiency rickets requiring hospital admission over a 30 month period, Dawodu and colleagues found and continue to find vitamin D deficiency, defined as serum 25(OH)D < 10 ng/ml, in 92% of the rachitic children and in 97% of their mothers (Dawodu et al., 2003; Dawodu & Wagner, 2007; Saadi et al., 2007). In the summer months in this sunny area in infants of Arab and South Asian ethnicity, investigators found serum 25(OH)D < 10 ng/ml in 61% of lactating mothers and in 82% of their children, demonstrating the prevalence of vitamin D deficiency in certain populations despite the availability of sun exposure (Dawodu et al., 2003).

Another study carried out in Australia reiterated the now, expectedly high prevalence of vitamin D deficiency in mothers of infants with rickets (Nozza & Rodda, 2001). In another study conducted in Greece, when summer-born infants and their mothers received no vitamin D supplementation, the infants exhibited mean serum 25(OH)D of 13.3 ng/mL at 6 months of age in the winter (Challa et al., 2005; Lapatsanis et al., 2005). These infants had a mean 25(OH)D concentration of 10.1 ng/mL at 1 postnatal week, showing the inadequacy of the reserves created during summer months to maintain sufficient stores of vitamin D metabolites to avoid vitamin D deficiency. These reports highlighted the need to provide a more universal and time-honored vitamin D supplementation dose that not only would prevent rickets, but the other potential long-latency disease states we now associate with vitamin D deficiency (Wagner & Greer, 2008).

Gessner et al. reported in 2003 on the prevalence of vitamin D deficiency among infants and young children in Alaska: 11% of healthy 6- to 23-month-old children in Alaska had circulating 25(OH)D levels <15 ng/mL (<37 nmol/L) and 20% had concentrations 37 to 62 nmol/L (Gessner, deSchweinitz, Petersen, & Lewandowski, 1997; Gessner, Plotnik, & Muth, 2003), with the lowest levels seen in those infants who were breastfeeding. After this study, the Alaska Special Supplemental Nutrition Program for Women, Infants, and Children (WIC) began an initiative to actively identify breastfeeding children and provide free vitamin D supplements for them and a vitamin D fact sheet for their mothers.

Another study in a more southern region of the United States—as compared to Alaska—conducted by Ziegler et al., assessed the vitamin D status of 84 breastfeeding infants in Iowa (latitude 41°N) (Ziegler, Hollis, Nelson, & Jeter, 2006). In this study, 10% of breastfeeding infants at 9 months of age had serum 25(OH)D levels < 11 ng/ml (profound deficiency) with most deficiency noted during winter months, with darker skin pigmentation, and in those who received no vitamin D supplement. Specifically, in this group of 87 breastfed infants, only 5% received vitamin D supplementation. In the 34 infants who received no supplemental vitamin D, 8 infants (23%) had a serum 25(OH)D concentration 11 ng/mL (<27 nmol/L) at 280 days of age. Seven of eight of these low measurements were made in the winter months (November through April).

Ziegler et al.'s study in the United States demonstrates the high prevalence of vitamin D deficiency, even in a country with vitamin D fortification of milk products and recommendations for infant and nursing mother vitamin D supplementation (Wagner & Greer, 2008). Studies such as those by Dawodu (Dawodu et al., 2003; Dawodu & Tsang, 2007; Dawodu & Wagner, 2007; Saadi et al., 2007), Gessner (Gessner et al., 1997; Gessner et al., 2003), Ziegler (Ziegler et al., 2006) and others, which highlight the pervasiveness of vitamin D deficiency in multiple settings, reinforce the need for vitamin D supplementation in infants and children that take into consideration latitude, season, skin pigmentation, culture, and clothing practices to promote adequate vitamin D status for the health of all infants.

Use of Vitamin D Supplementation in Neonates, Infants and Young Children

In 1963, the American Academy of Pediatrics (AAP) made its first recommendation of vitamin D supplementation in infants and children of 400 IU/day (Academy of Pediatrics, 1963). This amount continued to be the recommended supplementation dose for infants and children until the AAP, in accordance with the Institute of Medicine's recommendations (Standing Committee on Dietary Reference Intakes, 1997), revised its recommendation in 2003 and lowered the recommended dose to 200 IU/day (Gartner et al., 2003) for all breastfed infants within the first 2 months of life, at a time when breastfeeding was well established (Gartner et al., 2003).

The change was based principally on data from the United States, Norway, and China showing that 200 IU of vitamin D would prevent physical signs of vitamin D deficiency, i.e., rickets, as well as maintain 25(OH)D levels in what was considered to be the sufficient range at the time—11 ng/mL or 27.5 nmol/L (Gartner et al., 2003). The revised recommendations relied heavily on data from a prospective study conducted in four locations in China that demonstrated no evidence of rickets at 6 months in infants receiving as low as 100 IU per day vitamin D supplementation (Specker et al., 1992). Since rickets has been clinically apparent with circulating 25(OH)D concentrations below 11 ng/ml, this level is commonly considered to define vitamin D deficiency in infants (Gartner et al., 2003). Yet, as we have learned, the absence of rickets is not a surrogate for vitamin D sufficiency: despite the absence of overt rickets in this cohort, over 30% of the infants in the Northern locations had circulating 25(OH)D concentrations below 11 ng/ml (Specker et al., 1992).

Since the 2003 AAP revised recommendations, the wisdom of that limited supplementation dose has been called into question with continued reports of vitamin D deficiency and rickets reported in infants and young children throughout the world (Nozza & Rodda, 2001; Challa et al., 2005; Dawodu et al., 2005; Lapatsanis et al., 2005; Ziegler et al., 2006; Dawodu & Tsang, 2007; Dawodu & Wagner, 2007; Ward et al., 2007). Interestingly, after the 2003 revised AAP recommendations, United States formula companies did not change formula vitamin D content, which continue to provide to this day at least 400 IU/L (Atkinson & Tsang, 2005). Thus, an exclusively formula-fed infant over 1 month of age commonly will drink at least a liter of formula per day, which will provide a minimum of 400 IU vitamin D to that infant per day, without reports of vitamin D toxicity. In addition, the infant vitamin supplement readily available in the United States continues to provide a standard dose of 400 IU/day (Mead Johnson, 2004). Also, remember that 1 teaspoon of cod liver oil was recommended for infants and children to prevent rickets (Guy, 1923; Cannell et al., 2008); as we discussed earlier, 1 teaspoon of cod liver oil happens to contain around 400 IU vitamin D_3. With the exception of children with Williams Syndrome (Knudtzon, Aksnes, Akslen, & Aarskog, 1987; Mathias, 2000; Aravena et al., 2002), 400 IU vitamin D per day is safe for neonates, infants, and children (Academy of Pediatrics, 1963)

Treatment of infants and children to prevent vitamin D deficiency is different than treatment of infants and children with evidence of actual severe vitamin D deficiency and/or rickets, as the first approach is prevention and the second is treatment to correct an already detected abnormality or disease state. Gordon et al. (2008) published their findings of vitamin D supplementation in infants and young children with evidence of hypovitaminosis D (as defined by a circulating 25(OH)D level <20 ng/mL). They compared three oral vitamin D treatment regimens: daily vitamin D_2, weekly vitamin D_2, and daily vitamin D_3. They found that each of the three treatments more than tripled circulating 25(OH)D levels in the infants and children, and that there were no differences, however, between daily vs. weekly vitamin D_2 or in daily vitamin D_2 vs. D_3. These results suggest that a vitamin D supplementation regimen that is most suitable for the patient should be adopted. In a related study, Soliman et al. (2010) administered a single 10,000 IU/kg intramuscular dose of vitamin D_3 to infants and toddlers living in Qatar with vitamin-D-deficient rickets (as defined by low serum 25(OH)D, elevated alkaline phosphatase with clinical manifestation of rickets). There was no evidence of toxicity with this regimen noted. While the single intramuscular injection did not attain a consistent increase in circulating 25(OH)D to above 20 ng/mL (4/40 or 10% had levels <10 ng/mL) at 6 months post treatment, 38/40 (95%) had resolution of bony changes on X-ray. This approach and that of Gordon et al. (2008) may be utilized in those patients where adherence to a regimen, such as daily vitamin D supplementation or even weekly supplementation, may not be followed.

Once you have chosen a particular vitamin D regimen, how do you sort out which preparation to use? Clearly, vitamin D has been given along with other vitamins in a multivitamin preparation that is safe and cost-effective. Yet, to the breastfeeding mother, giving additional vitamins that are not deemed necessary may be unacceptable. Vitamin D-only preparations have come on the market during the past 5 years, including those available as a single drop. **Table 3** summarizes the commercially available vitamin D preparations that are currently on the market.

Table 3. Oral Vitamin D Preparations Currently Available in the United States (in Alphabetical Order)

Preparation	Dosage[15]
Baby Ddrops™ The Ddrops Company Toronto, Canada www.ddrops.ca (distributed in U.S. through Carlson Labs)	1 drop gives 400 IU Coconut and palm oil preparation Also comes in 2,000 IU/drop preparation Five-year shelf life
Bio-D-Mulsion™ Biotics Research Laboratory Rosenberg, Texas www.bioticsresearch.com	1 drop gives 400 IU Corn oil preparation Also comes in 2,000 IU/drop preparation** One-year shelf life
Just D™ Sunlight Vitamins, Inc.	1 mL gives 400 IU Corn oil preparation
Carlson Laboratories www.carlsonlabs.com	1 gel cap gives 400 IU Also comes in 2,000 IU gel caps**
Multivitamin preparations polyvitamins A, D, and K vitamin preparations	1 mL gives 400 IU

Adapted from the AAP Statement (Wagner, Greer, et al., 2008). Reproduced with permission from Pediatrics, 133(5), ©2008 by AAP.

[15] Note: Higher-dose oral preparations may be necessary for the treatment of those with rickets in the first few months of therapy or for patients with chronic diseases, such as fat malabsorption (cystic fibrosis), or patients chronically taking medications that interfere with vitamin D metabolism (such as antiseizure medications).

Because a single drop regimen's effectiveness had not been previously tested in infants, practitioners have had some trepidation in using such a preparation. Using an oil emulsion preparation, we sought to measure its effectiveness in our ongoing lactation trial (Wagner, Howard, et al., 2010). As part of a larger, ongoing vitamin D supplementation trial of fully lactating women, infants of mothers assigned to the control group received 400 IU vitamin D_3 in 1 drop per day dosing starting at 1 month of age. Subjects were enrolled throughout the year. As part of our data safety and monitoring process, infant 25(OH)D levels (mean ± S.D.) were measured by radioimmunoassay at visits 1 (~1 month of age; baseline), 4, and 7. Fifty-four mothers and their infants were enrolled in the study and randomized to the control group in a blinded fashion; 33 completed the study through visit 7. The mean ± S.D. 25(OH)D at 1 month (baseline) for the infants was 16.0 ± 9.3 ng/mL (range 1.0-40.8; n=33). The mean levels increased to 43.6 ± 14.1 (range 18.2-69.7) at 4 months and remained relatively unchanged at month 7: 42.5 ± 12.1 ng/mL (range 18.9-67.2). The change in values between 1 and 4 months, and 1 and 7 months was statistically significant (p≤0.0001). As predicted, there were no statistically significant differences between months 4 and 7 (p=0.66). Even with changes in season, the results remained significant.

Of note, despite the decrease in dose on a per kilogram basis, the infant mean circulating 25(OH)D levels were not significantly different between visit 4 and 7: at visit 1, the infants were receiving 88.9 ± 10.5 IU/kg; at visit 4, they were receiving 59.7 ± 6.6 IU/kg; and at visit 7, they were receiving 50.5 ± 6.0 IU/kg (p<0.0001) (Wagner, Howard, et al., 2010). Overall, the infant's circulating 25(OH)D levels increased 37% above baseline. There were no adverse events associated with the prescribed vitamin D supplementation. While not powered to assess safety at this juncture, it is important to note that, thus far, there have been no increased rates of

a A study by Martínez et al., (2006) showed that newborn and older infants preferred oil-based liquid preparations to alcohol-based preparations.

b Single-drop preparation may be better tolerated in patients with oral aversion issues, but proper instruction regarding administration of these drops must be given to the parents or care provider, given the increased risk of toxicity, incorrect dosing, or accidental ingestion.

c The cost of vitamin D–only preparations may be more than multivitamin preparations and could be an issue for health clinics that dispense vitamins to infants and children. The multivitamin preparation was the only preparation available until recently; therefore, there is a comfort among practitioners in dispensing multivitamins to all age groups.

infection in the infants or adverse health effects that could be attributed to vitamin D supplementation in this cohort. Thus, oral vitamin D_3 supplementation as an oil emulsion (400 IU/drop) was associated with significant and sustained increases in circulating 25(OH)D from baseline in fully breastfeeding infants through 7 months of age.

In general, concerns about dosing infants with any medication, particularly as a single drop, are warranted-and remain so. The greatest risk appears to be if a parent is not instructed on how to give a medication or does not receive the full instruction on proper dispensing. We have found in our study of lactating women that demonstrating how to give the drop to be the best method of teaching proper dispensing. Mothers are asked to demonstrate how to give the drop prior to leaving the research outpatient clinic, and this method has been found to be effective. Whatever method is prescribed by the health care professional, caution must be exhibited and an assessment of how well a prescription is understood must be made. This approach will ensure the safety of that patient—in this case—the newborn, infant, or young child.

What Are the Latest Recommendations?

This is a moving target. As more research is published, we have a better understanding of both the vitamin D requirements of the lactating mother and her recipient infant and the safety of higher doses of vitamin D. Based on available data; the recommendations are a work in progress. When asked the question, what is the effect of such maternal deficiency on her infant?—we can unequivocally state—**deficiency, of course**. In comparison, what is the effect of maternal vitamin D sufficiency on the breastfeeding infant?—**Sufficiency, of course**. Thus, the status of the mother and that of her breastfeeding infant are intertwined: they are a mirror of each other (Hillman & Haddad, 1974; Moncrieff & Fadahunsi, 1974; Rosen, Roginsky, Nathenson, & Finberg, 1974; Hollis & Wagner, 2004b; Wagner et al., 2006).

Infant deficiency is more apparent to the eye because the infant shows physical signs and symptoms of vitamin D deficiency much more readily than the adult—in the form of rickets. Yet, as has been discussed in this and earlier sections, rickets is really just one of the many sequelae of vitamin D deficiency (Liu et al., 2006; Holick,

2007a). Current studies investigating the role of vitamin D in maintaining health goes well beyond bone and calcium metabolism to the realm of acute infection and long-latency diseases that are linked by vitamin D's role in the immune system (Lefkowitz & Garland, 1994; Boucher, Mannan, Noonan, Hales, & Evans, 1995; Hypponen et al., 2001; Krall, Wehler, Garcia, Harris, & Dawson-Hughes, 2001; Looker, Dawson-Hughes, Calvo, Gunter, & Sahyoun, 2002; Borissova et al., 2003; Bischoff-Ferrari et al., 2004; Chiu et al., 2004; Dawson-Hughes, Heaney, Holick, Lips, Meunier, & Vieth, 2004; Dietrich, Joshipura, Dawson-Hughes, & Bischoff-Ferrari, 2004; Hypponen, 2004; Hypponen et al., 2004; Munger et al., 2004; Dietrich, Nunn, Dawson-Hughes, & Bisfchoff-Ferrari, 2005; Giovannucci, 2005; Harris, 2005; Hypponen, 2005; Whiting & Calvo, 2005; Bischoff-Ferrari, Giovannucci, Willett, Dietrich, & Dawson-Hughes, 2006; Cannell et al., 2006; Giovannucci et al., 2006; Munger et al., 2006; Giovannucci, 2007; Hypponen, Hartikainen, Sovio, Jarvelin, & Pouta, 2007; Hypponen & Power, 2007; Lappe, Travers-Gustafson, Davies, Recker, & Heaney, 2007; Pittas, Harris, Stark, & Dawson-Hughes, 2007; Pittas, Lau, et al., 2007). To really understand the requirements of the breastfeeding infant, one must understand how vitamin D from the mother is transferred to her recipient breastfeeding baby.

As we have shown, breastfed infants can maintain sufficient vitamin D status solely through adequate sunlight exposure (Ho et al., 1985; Specker, Valanis, et al., 1985), but the practicality and safety of extended sunlight exposure to achieve this is in question. There continue to be valid concerns regarding increased risk of certain skin cancers with repeated, chronic UV exposure (American Academy of Pediatrics, 1999). The recommendations to use sunscreen to prevent burning while outdoors are substantiated by the ever-growing rates of skin cancers (National Coalition for Skin Cancer Prevention, 1998; Greer, 2004); preventive measures, such as the use of sunscreens and protective barriers, makes adequate sun exposure for vitamin D synthesis unlikely in most infants (American Academy of Pediatrics, 1999; Wagner, Greer, & AAP, 2008). With the data that are available at this time, the only way to ensure adequate vitamin D status in the infant and child who is breastfeeding is to use an oral vitamin D supplement.

As mentioned earlier, concurrent with the AAP's 2003 vitamin D statement (Gartner et al., 2003), expanding information, mostly in adult literature, has linked vitamin

D insufficiency to other biochemical markers involved in bone mineralization, calcium absorption, insulin resistance, and innate immunity. In response to these findings, new definitions of vitamin D deficiency and insufficiency have developed. For adults, vitamin D deficiency is now defined as a total circulating (or serum) 25(OH)D level < 20 ng/mL or 50 nmol/L, and vitamin D insufficiency as a total circulating 25(OH)D level in the range of 20 ng/mL or 50 nmol/L to 32 ng/mL or 80 nmol/L; therefore, vitamin D sufficiency is defined as a circulating 25(OH)D level of 32 ng/mL or 80 nmol/L. As a result, concerns rose regarding the adequacy of supplementation of infants with only 200 IU of vitamin D, and the question of normal vitamin D status in infants and children was raised (Taylor, Wagner, & Hollis, 2008; Wagner, Greer, et al. 2008; Wagner, Taylor, & Hollis, 2008).

Because of the paucity of data on the subject, definitive ranges for infants and children have yet to be declared, but research has shown that in today's living conditions, supplementation with 200 IU/day of vitamin D is inadequate to achieve circulating 25(OH)D levels > 20 ng/mL or 50 nmol/L. The time-honored use of 1 teaspoon of cod liver oil, which supplied 400 IU, has served as a model to suggest that supplementation with 400 IU/day of vitamin D is adequate to achieve circulating 25(OH)D levels of at least 20 ng/mL or 50 nmol/L (Pittard et al., 1991; Wagner et al., 2006; Wagner, Greer, et al. 2008). Further, this premise is based on the following well established facts:

(1) Vitamin D deficiency can occur early in life, particularly when many pregnant women themselves are deficient (Hollis & Wagner, 2004a; Hollis & Wagner, 2004b; Basile et al., 2007).

(2) Serum 25(OH)D levels of unsupplemented breastfed infants often are <20 ng/mL (50 nmol/L), particularly in winter months and latitudes farther from the equator, likely secondary to maternal deficiency.

(3) Adequate sunlight exposure in a given infant to achieve adequate vitamin D synthesis is difficult to determine and often not achieved (Wagner & Greer, 2008).

(4) Serum 25(OH)D levels can be maintained > 20 ng/mL or 50 nmol/L in breastfed infants with supplementation of 400 IU/day of vitamin D (Wagner & Greer, 2008; Wagner, Greer, et al. 2008).

In light of these observations, the AAP recently amended its previous recommendation for vitamin D supplementation of infants and children (Wagner & Greer, 2008). The current recommendation reads:

> *A supplement of 400 IU/day of vitamin D should begin within the first few days of life and continue throughout childhood. Any breastfeeding infant, regardless of whether he or she is being supplemented with formula, should be supplemented with 400 IU of vitamin D (p. 1142).*

Vitamin D preparations either in vitamin D-only or multi-vitamin supplements are readily available and inexpensive.

As human milk has repeatedly been reaffirmed as the ideal nutrition for infants' healthy growth and development with the exception of inadequate concentrations of vitamin D, the ideal situation would be to improve the nutritional status of the human milk to avoid the need for any supplementation. Early investigation to improve maternal vitamin D status, thereby improving the nutritional status of her milk, are promising, but a well established dose to achieve this goal has not yet been established. In addition, we know that vitamin D insufficiency affects multiple organ systems, including the immune system, bone mineralization, and cardiovascular system based upon adult literature, but the long-term implications for fetuses and infants developing in a vitamin insufficient state have not been studied. The question remains: how does vitamin D insufficiency, and frank deficiency, during early embryogenesis and into infancy impact the innate programming for adult disease? In order to answer this question and those like it, further vitamin D research is needed, particularly in the areas of pregnancy, lactation, and long-term consequences for the infant.

Maternal vitamin D deficiency and the resulting nutritional rickets in her nursing infant is a preventable disorder whose occurrence has increased during the last two decades. Through careful research, we understand more fully that this deficiency is not caused by something that is inherently "wrong" or "missing" in mother's milk, but rather by suboptimal maternal vitamin D status and the resultant low concentrations in the mother's milk.

As new evidence points to serious consequences of chronic vitamin D deprivation, including decreased bone mass in later life, as well as increased risks of periodontal disease, infections, Type-I diabetes, neoplasia, myopathy, and depression, we must establish normative guidelines for safe and effective vitamin D supplementation during lactation in both the lactating woman *and* her infant that address modern-day lifestyles. Through the ongoing and unfolding discovery that with sufficient vitamin D supplementation of the mother, human milk can provide adequate vitamin D supply to the nursing infant, we are experiencing what pediatrician and breastfeeding expert Dr. Ruth Lawrence refers to as "shifting the vitamin D paradigm" (Lawrence, 2008). This shift supports both the lactating woman and her breastfeeding infant by reestablishing the premise that human milk is truly a complete nutritional and bioactive substance for the breastfeeding infant. "It is clear that, at least in part, vitamin D does make the world go 'round' " (Wagner, Taylor, & Hollis, 2008, p. 246).

12. Vitamin D Recommendations for the Pregnant and Lactating Woman and her Infant

As we discussed earlier, the recommendations for vitamin D requirements have changed during the past century as the views of vitamin D's role in metabolism and toxicity have changed. It is a work in progress and each new study that helps us ascertain vitamin D's function within the body in various systems through the lifespan challenges our notion of what is required to reach optimal levels, processing, and function within. There have been extensive data to suggest that vitamin D supplementation of 400 IU/day during the first year of life is adequate, but whether that amount is optimal remains to be proved. As the child grows, on a per kilogram basis, 400 IU/day is likely insufficient beyond a year, especially in those children with limited milk intake and sunlight exposure, in those with darker pigmentation, and who live at higher latitudes.

Conjecture continues and at the heart of all of this is the notable concern that we do not succumb to what other generations have seen—a little is good and a lot is better. The countercurrent or rebound of the pendulum will as quickly and decisively swing in the other direction, and we will be worse than we ever were, with rampant deficiency replaced by toxicity. We have reviewed what is known about toxicity as it exists today with the limited food fortifications. We know that compliance with any medication or supplement varies, depending on the motivation of that individual and the perception that the particular medicine or supplement is really necessary. There are those who will follow any recommendation to the letter, those who will not follow it all, those who follow it variably, and finally, those who will follow any recommendation and double or triple it. Acetaminophen is an excellent example of this. As we gain greater experience with a certain medication or supplement, that experience is enriched by the ability to monitor a metabolite of that medication or supplement that furthers our comfort level. This is as true for vitamin D as any other medication or supplement.

One size does *not*, nor will it ever, fit everyone. Variability in where one lives, one's diet, one's lifestyle, one's body composition (fat mass and lean body mass), and the season affect one's final vitamin D status. When we say, "with all things being equal," we are talking about lab animals or clones of individuals who do not exist in the real world. With all that being said, what does one do? The solution is that there must be a range of supplementation that will be safe and effective for a vast number of individuals of that given age, gender, or weight class. There also must be refinement of what we hold true today based on the rigors of scientific investigation and evidence—evidence that makes physiological sense and stands true with the test of time. We tend to ignore those findings which show flaws in our thinking, in our data. We would not find ourselves in this predicament of overwhelming vitamin D deficiency had we applied this wisdom and scrutinized what we held to be irrefutable. It is uncanny that the very same data used and interpreted differently by the scientific camp in which one lives—those who see vitamin D as a (prepro)hormone that must be provided in adequate quantity for all ages and sizes and those who fear toxicity and the unknown of "lifting the ban on vitamin D" are looking at the same "evidence." One thing is clear, however, and it is that there are many who hold neither view, but exist with their beliefs somewhere in the middle. Those of us who have studied vitamin D and seen the ravage of deficiency on physiology lean to the left and our defense is our science and our data that have stood up to the naysayer light.

With these caveats in mind, we can ask the question yet again: what should one do when it comes to vitamin D? The answer is found in **Table 4**:

Table 4. Suggested Vitamin D Supplementation Regimen for Pregnant and Lactating Women, Infants, Children

Age Group	Recommended Daily Vitamin D Intake (IU/day)	Caveats to Ponder
Neonates	400 IU/day	This includes premature neonates and infants. More data are needed to determine what the IU/kg requirements are of preterm infants and neonates born to mothers with frank vitamin D deficiency
Infants < 1 year	400 IU/day up to 10 kg; then 25-50 IU/kg	
Children 1-2 yrs	25-50 IU/kg	For example, a child weighing 20 kg would be given 500-1,000 IU/day. Another child weighing 25 kg would be given 625-1,250 IU/day. One could give the lower dose during summer months and the higher dose during winter months.
Children 2-5 years	25-50 IU/kg up to 30 kg	
Children 5-12 years	25 IU/kg up to 50 kg	
Children 12-17 years	>50 kg	2,000-4,000 IU/day depending on BMI
Pregnant woman	>45 kg	4,000 IU vitamin D/day [This recommendation is based on our two RCT that were completed in 2009 (Wagner, Johnson, et al., 2010; Wagner, McNeil, et al., 2010).]
Lactating Woman		Likely 6.400 IU/day with refinement of recommendation once Lactation RCT vitamin D studies have been completed and analyzed.

This is a conservative guide. If an individual has an increased BMI or a history of malabsorption, then that individual may require higher daily vitamin D supplementation. It would be prudent to check levels if increasing intake beyond these recommendations. The ultimate goal is to attain circulating 25(OH)D levels in that individual that would mimic living in a sun-rich environment with daily sun exposure.

Children would receive incremental doses of vitamin D based on their weight and percent body fat to maintain circulating 25(OH)D levels, with a minimum of 32 ng/mL or 80 nmol/L. Those children and teenagers with higher BMI's will require higher daily vitamin D intake to achieve a circulating 25(OH)D level of at least 32 ng/mL. Latitude, skin pigmentation, sunlight exposure and sunscreen use, and BMI are all factors that must be taken into account when making recommendations concerning vitamin D supplementation.

Pregnant women would be encouraged to take 4,000 IU/day and lactating women at least 4000 IU/day, with the expected increase in the recommendation once studies with lactating women and their infants have been completed. Our experience thus far has been that doses of 6400 IU/day are necessary to raise maternal milk vitamin D levels in the adequate range, so that the infant is ingesting at least 400 IU/L breastmilk. While the efficacy of this dosing regimen has been tested, the **safety of this regimen has not been fully tested in a large cohort of women**. On an individual basis, if a health care professional prescribes higher doses to a lactating woman, it is recommended that the woman's breastfeeding infant have levels checked to ensure that the baby is vitamin D replete. Alternatively, giving a lactating woman sufficient vitamin D to achieve a level of at least 80 nmol/L or 32 ng/mL could be complemented with infant oral supplementation of a vitamin D-only preparation containing 400 IU per measured volume to be given daily. This is the standard of care at this time in the U.S., with 800 IU/day recommended for those living above latitude 45°N.

In the end, it is not sufficient to accept marginal vitamin D status, just as one would not accept or support marginal status of other hormones, such as thyroxine in someone with hypothyroidism. As is the case with every hormone or preprohormone/hormone system, we prescribe a regimen to correct the hormonal deficiency and we do not hesitate to check a follow-up level. While not discussed in any real detail in this book, the measurement of the nutritional indicator of vitamin D—namely, total circulating 25(OH)D is a fastidious and exacting process. One must ensure that the laboratory that is used has independent validation of the levels reported. Once optimal vitamin D status and how to achieve it has been determined throughout the lifespan, there will be less need to check levels. We will "know" through experience that 4,000 IU vitamin D/day does the "trick" for the pregnant woman, just as we know today that 400 IU vitamin D/day does the "trick" in preventing rickets and other health sequelae in infants during the first year of life. Our learning curve is steep and we have come a long way since 1999 when Dr. Vieth first wowed the world with his "heretical" high-dose vitamin D safety trial (Vieth, 1999). We continue to build on the exacting rigors of scientific inquiry into the realm of vitamin D, and we should continue to demand nothing less. In the end, we must take the time to appreciate that the needs of our patients may not fit the schema that we have been taught, but rather here before us is a challenge that will help us to better understand and redefine what is really science and medicine at its finest—discovery. It is through such discovery and positive inquiry that we will redefine the vitamin D requirements during the 21st century.

REFERENCES

Abe, E., Miyaura, C., Sakagami, H., Takeda, M., Konno, K., Yamazaki, T., et al. (1981). Differentiation of mouse myeloid leukemia cells induced by 1 alpha,25-dihydroxyvitamin D_3. *Proceedings of the National Academy of Sciences of the United States of America, 78*(8), 4990-4994.

Acharya, A. B., Annamali, S., Taub, N. A., & Field, D. (2004). Oral sucrose analgesia for preterm infant venepuncture. *Archives of Disease in Childhood. Fetal and Neonatal Edition, 89*(1), F17-18.

Adams, J., & Gacad, M. (1985). Characterization of 1-a-hydroxylation of vitamin D_3 sterols by cultured alveolar macrophages from patients with sarcoidosis. *The Journal of Experimental Medicine, 161* 755-765.

Adams, J. S. (1989). Vitamin D metabolite-mediated hypercalcemia. *Endocrinology and Metabolism Clinics of North America, 18*(3), 765-778.

Adams, J. S., Clements, T. L., Parrish, J. A., & Holick, M. F. (1982). Vitamin D synthesis and metabolism after ultraviolet irradiation of normal and vitamin D-deficient subjects. *The New England Journal of Medicine, 306*, 722-725.

Adams, J. S., Fernandez, M., Gacad, M. A., Gill, P. S., Endres, D. B., Rasheed, S., et al. (1989). Vitamin D metabolite-mediated hypercalcemia and hypercalciuria patients with AIDS- and non-AIDS-associated lymphoma. *Blood, 73*(1), 235-239.

Akeno, N., Saikatsu, S., & Horiuchi, N. (1993). Increase of renal 25-hydroxyvitamin D_3-24-hydroxylase activity and its messenger ribonucleic acid level in 1 alpha-hydroxyvitamin D_3-administered rats: possibility of the presence of two forms of 24-hydroxylase. *Journal of Nutritional Science and Vitaminology (Tokyo), 39*(2), 89-100.

Akiba, T., Endou, H., Koseki, C., Sakai, F., Horiuchi, N., & Suda, T. (1980). Localization of 25-hydroxyvitamin D_3-1 alpha-hydroxylase activity in the mammalian kidney. *Biochemical and Biophysical Research Communications, 94*(1), 313-318.

Ala-Houhala, M. (1985). 25(OH)D levels during breast-feeding with or without maternal or infantile supplementation of vitamin D. *Journal of Pediatric Gastroenterology and Nutrition, 4*, 220-226.

Ala-Houhala, M., Koskinen, T., Parviainen, M., & Visakorpi, J. (1988). 25-Hydroxyvitamin D and vitamin D in human milk: effects of supplementation and season. *The American Journal of Clinical Nutrition, 48*(4), 1057-1060.

Ala-Houhala, M., Koskinen, T., Terho, A., Koivula, T., & Visakorpi, J. (1986). Maternal compared with infant vitamin D supplementation. *Archives of Disease in Childhood, 61*, 1159-1163.

Allgrove, J. (2009). Physiology of calcium, phosphate and magnesium. In J. Allgrove & N. J. Shaw, (Eds.), *Endocrine Development. Calcium and bone disorders in children and adolescents* (Vol. 16, pp. 8-31). Basel: Karger.

Alouf, B., & Grigalonis, M. (2005). Incidental finding of vitamin D deficient rickets in an otherwise healthy infant--a reappraisal of current vitamin-D supplementation guidelines. *Journal of the National Medical Association, 97*(8), 1170-1173.

American Academy of Pediatrics. Committee on Nutrition. (1963). *The prophylactic requirement and the toxicity of vitamin D.*

American Academy of Pediatrics. (1999).Policy Statement. Ultraviolet light: A hazard to children (RE9913). *Pediatrics, 104*(2), 328-333.

Anderson, D., & Schlesinger, B. (1940). Paper presented at the Society for Pediatric Research.

Antia, A. V., Wiltse, H. E., Rowe, R. D., Pitt, E. L., Levin, S., Ottesen, O. E., et al. (1967). Pathogenesis of the supravalvular aortic stenosis syndrome. *The Journal of Pediatrics, 71*, 431-441.

Arabian, A., Grover, J., Barre, M. G., & Delvin, E. E. (1993). Rat kidney 25-hydroxyvitamin D$_3$ 1 alpha- and 24-hydroxylases: evidence for two distinct gene products. *The Journal of Steroid Biochemistry and Molecular Biology, 45*(6), 513-516.

Aravena, T., Castillo, S., Carrasco, X., Mena, I., Lopez, J., Rojas, J. P., et al. (2002). Williams syndrome: clinical, cytogenetical, neurophysiological and neuroanatomic study. *Revista Médica de Chile, 130*, 631-637.

Argao, E., Heubi, J., Hollis, B., & Tsang, R. (1992). d-alpha-tocopheryl polyethylene glycol-1000 succinate enhances the absorption of vitamin D in chronic cholestatic liver disease of infancy and childhood. *Pediatric Research, 31*(2), 146-150.

Aris, R., Merkel, P., Bachrach, L., Borowitz, D., Boyle, M., Elkin, S., et al. (2005). Guide to bone health and disease in cystic fibrosis. *The Journal of Clinical Endocrinology and Metabolism, 90*(3), 1888-1896.

Armas, L., Hollis, B. W., & Heaney, R. P. (2004). Vitamin D$_2$ is much less effective than vitamin D$_3$ in humans. *The Journal of Clinical Endocrinology and Metabolism, 89*, 5387-5391.

Arnson, Y., Amital, H., & Shoenfeld, Y. (2007). Vitamin D and autoimmunity: new aetiological and therapeutic considerations, *Annals of the Rheumatic Diseases, 66*(9), 1137-1142).

Atkinson, S., & Tsang, R. (2005). Calcium, magnesium, phosphorus, and vitamin D. In R. Tsang, R. Uauy, B. Koletzko & S. Zlotkin (Eds.), *Nutrition of the Preterm Infant: Scientific Basis and Practical Guidelines* (2nd ed., pp. 245-276). Cincinnati: Digital Educational Publishing, Inc.

Bachrach, S., Fisher, J., & Parks, J. S. (1979). An outbreak of vitamin D deficiency rickets in a susceptible population. *Pediatrics, 64*, 871-877.

Baggenstoss, A., & Keith, H. (1941). Calcification of the arteries of an infant. Report of a case. *The Journal of Pediatrics, 18*, 95-102.

Bahr, G. M., Eales, L. J., Nye, K. E., Majeed, H. A., Yousof, A. M., Behbehani, K., et al. (1989). An association between Gc (vitamin D-binding protein) alleles and susceptibility to rheumatic fever. *Immunology, 67*(1), 126-128.

Baker, A. R., McDonnell, D. P., Hughes, M., Crisp, T. M., Mangelsdorf, D. J., Haussler, M. R., et al. (1988). Cloning and expression of full-length cDNA encoding human vitamin D receptor. *Proceedings of the National Academy of Sciences of the United States of America, 85*(10), 3294-3298.

Balasubramanian, S., Shivbalan, S., & Kumar, P. S. (2006). Hypocalcemia due to vitamin D deficiency in exclusively breastfed infants. *Indian Pediatrics, 43*(3), 247-251.

Bandeira, F., Griz, L., Dryer, P., Eufrazino, C., Bandeira, C., & Freese, E. (2006). Vitamin D deficiency: A global perspective. *Arquivos Brasileiros de Endocrinologia & Metabologia, 50*, 640-646.

Barragry, J., France, M., Corless, D., Gupta, S., Switals, S., Boucher, B., et al. (1978). Intestinal cholecalciferol absorption in the elderly and in younger adults. *Clinical Science and Molecular Medicine, 55*(2), 213-220.

Barragry, J. M., Corless, D., Auton, J., & et.al. (1978). Plasma vitamin D-binding globulin in vitamin D deficiency, pregnancy and chronic liver disease. *Clinica Chimica Acta, 87,* 359.

Barrueto, F., Jr., Wang-Flores, H. H., Howland, M. A., Hoffman, R. S., & Nelson, L. S. (2005). Acute Vitamin D Intoxication in a Child. *Pediatrics, 116*(3), e453-456.

Basile, L., Taylor, S., Quinones, L., Wagner, C., & Hollis, B. (2007). Neonatal vitamin D status at birth at latitude 32°72': Evidence of widespread deficiency. *Journal of Perinatology, 27*(9), 568-571.

Becker, A., Eyles, D., McGrath, J., & Grecksch, G. (2005). Transient prenatal vitamin D deficiency is associated with subtle alterations in learning and memory functions in adult rats. *Behavioural Brain Research, 161,* 306-312.

Becroft, D. M. O., & Chambers, D. (1976). Supravalvular aortic stenosis-infantile hypercalcemia syndrome: *in vitro* hypersensitivitiy to vitamin D and calcium. *Journal of Medical Genetics, 13,* 223-228.

Bell, N. H., Shaw, S., & Turner, R. T. (1984). Evidence that 1,25-dihydroxyvitamin D_3 inhibits the hepatic production of 25-hydroxyvitamin D in man. *The Journal of Clinical Investigation, 74*(4), 1540-1544.

Bhattacharyya, M. H., & Deluca, H. F. (1974). Subcellular location of rat liver calciferol-25-hydroxylase. *Archives of Biochemistry and Biophysics, 160,* 58-62.

Bikle, D., Adams, J., & Christakos, S. (2008). Vitamin D: production, metabolism, mechanism of action, and clinical requirements. In C. Rosen (Ed.), *Primer on the metabolic bone diseases and disorders of mineral metabolism* (7th ed., pp. 141-149). Washington, DC: American Society for Bone and Mineral Research.

Bikle, D. D., Gee, E., Halloran, B. P., & et.al. (1986). Assessment of free fractions of 25-hydroxyvitamin D in serum and its regulation by albumin and vitamin D-binding protein. *The Journal of Clinical Endocrinology and Metabolism, 63,* 954.

Binet, A., & Kooh, S. W. (1996). Persistence of Vitamin D-deficiency rickets in Toronto in the 1990s. *Canadian Journal of Public Health, 87*(4), 227-230.

Bischoff-Ferrari, H., Dietrich, T., Orav, E., & Dawson-Hughes, B. (2004). Positive association between 25(OH)D levels and bone mineral density: A population-based study of younger and older adults. *The American Journal of Medicine, 116,* 634-639.

Bischoff-Ferrari, H., Giovannucci, E., Willett, W., Dietrich, T., & Dawson-Hughes, B. (2006). Estimation of optimal serum concentrations of 25-hydroxyvitamin D for multiple health outcomes. *The American Journal of Clinical Nutrition, 84,* 18-28.

Bjorkhem, I., & Holmberg, I. (1978). Assay and properties of a mitochondrial 25-hydroxylase active on vitamine D_3. *The Journal of Biological Chemistry, 253*(3), 842-849.

Black, J., & Bonham-Carter, J. (1963). Association between aortic stenosis and facies of severe infantile hypercalcemia. *Lancet, 2,* 745-749.

Blumberg, R., Forbes, G., & Fraser, D. (1963). The prophylactic requirement and the toxicity of vitamin D. *Pediatrics, 31,* 512-525.

Boris, A., Hurley, J. F., & Trmal, T. (1977). Relative activities of some metabolites and analogs of cholecalciferol in stimulation of tibia ash weight in chicks otherwise deprived of vitamin D. *The Journal of Nutrition, 107*(2), 194-198.

Borissova, A. M., Tankova, T., Kirilov, G., Dakovska, L., & Kovacheva, R. (2003). The effect of vitamin D_3 on insulin secretion and peripheral insulin sensitivity in type 2 diabetic patients. *International Journal of Clinical Practice, 57*(4), 258-261.

Boucher, B. J. (1995). Strategies for reduction in the prevalence of NIDDM; the case for a population-based approach to the development of policies to deal with environmental factors in its aetiology. *Diabetologia, 38*(9), 1125-1129.

Boucher, B. J., Mannan, N., Noonan, K., Hales, C. N., & Evans, S. J. (1995). Glucose intolerance and impairment of insulin secretion in relation to vitamin D deficiency in east London Asians. *Diabetologia, 38*(10), 1239-1245.

Bouillon, R., Van Assche, F. A., Van Baelen, H., Heyns, W., & DeMoor, P. (1981). Influence of the Vitamin D-binding protein on serum concentrations of $1,25(OH)_2D$. *The Journal of Clinical Investigation, 67*, 589-596.

Bouillon, R., Van Baelen, H., & DeMoor, D. (1977). 25-Hydroxy-vitamin D and its binding protein in maternal and cord serum. *The Journal of Clinical Endocrinology and Metabolism, 45*, 679-684.

Brockmann, H. (1936). Die Isolierung des antirachitischen Vitamins aus Thunfischleberol. *Hoppe-Seyler's Zeitschrift für Physiologische Chemie, 241*, 104-115.

Brooke, O. G., Brown, I. R. F., Bone, C. D. M., Carter, N. D., Cleeve, H. J. W., Maxwell, J. D., et al. (1980). Vitamin D supplements in pregnant Asian women: Effects on calcium status and fetal growth. *British Medical Journal, 1*, 751-754.

Brooke, O. G., Butters, F., & Wood, C. (1981). Intrauterine vitamin D nutrition and postnatal growth in Asian infants. *British Medical Journal, 283*, 1024.

Brown, E., & Hebert, S. (1997). Calcium-receptor-regulated parathyroid and renal function. *Bone, 20*(4), 303-309.

Brown, J., Bianco, J., McGrath, J., & Eyles, D. (2003). 1,25-Dihydroxyvitamin D-3 induces nerve growth factor, promotes neurite outgrowth and inhibits mitosis in embryonic rat hippocampal neurons. . *Neuroscience Letters, 343*, 139-143.

Brunvand, L., Haga, P., Tangsrud, S. E., & Haug, E. (1995). Congestive heart failure caused by vitamin D deficiency? *Acta Paediatrica, 84*, 1, 106-108.

Brunvard, L., Quigstad, E., Urdal, P., & Haug, E. (1996). Vitamin D deficiency and fetal growth. *Early Human Development, 45*, 27-33.

Burne, T., Becker, A., Brown, J., Eyles, D., MacKay-Sim, A., & McGrath, J. (2004). Transient prenatal vitamin D deficiency is associated with hyperlocomotion in adult rats. *Behavioral Brain Research, 154*, 549-555.

Burne, T., Feron, F., Brown, J., Eyles, D., McGrath, J., & Mackay-Sim, A. (2004). Combined prenatal and chronic postnatal vitamin D deficiency in rats impairs prepulse inhibition of acoustic startle. *Physiology & Behavior, 81*, 651-655.

Caicedo, R. A., Li, N., Atkinson, M. A., Schatz, D. A., & Neu, J. (2005). Neonatal Nutritional Interventions in the Prevention of Type 1 Diabetes. *Neoreviews, 6*(5), e220-226.

Cali, J. J., Hsieh, C. L., Francke, U., & Russell, D. W. (1991). Mutations in the bile acid biosynthetic enzyme sterol 27-hydroxylase underlie cerebrotendinous xanthomatosis. *The Journal of Biological Chemistry, 266*(12), 7779-7783.

Cancela, L., LeBoulch, N., & Miravet, L. (1986). Relationship between the vitamin D content of maternal milk and the vitamin D status of nursing women and breastfed infants. *The Journal of Endocrinology, 110*, 43-50.

Cannell, J. J., Vieth, R., Umhau, J. C., Holick, M. F., Grant, W. B., Madronich, S., et al. (2006). Epidemic influenza and vitamin D. *Epidemiology and Infection, 134*(6), 1129-1140.

Cannell, J. J., Vieth, R., Willett, W., Zasloff, M., Hathcock, J. N., White, J. H., et al. (2008). Cod liver oil, vitamin A toxicity, frequent respiratory infections, and the vitamin D deficiency epidemic. *The Annals of Otology, Rhinology, and Laryngology, 117*(11), 864-870.

Caverzasio, J., Montessuit, C., & Bonjour, J. (1990). Stimulatory effect of insulin-like growth factor-1 on renal Pi transport and plasma 1,25-dihydroxyvitamin D_3. *Endocrinology, 127*(1), 453-459.

Challa, A., Ntourntoufi, A., Cholevas, V., Bitsori, M., Galanakis, E., & Andronikou, S. (2005). Breastfeeding and vitamin D status in Greece during the first 6 months of life. *European Journal of Pediatrics, 164*(12), 724-729.

Chan, G. M., Buchino, D., Mehlhorn, K. E., Bove, K. E., Steichen, J. J., & Tsang, R. C. (1979). Effect of Vitamin D on Pregnant rabbits and their offspring. *Pediatric Research, 13*, 121-126.

Chapuy, M. C., Arlot, M., DuBoeuf, F., Brun, J., Crouzet, B., Arnaud, S., et al. (1992). Vitamin D_3 and calcium to prevent hip fractures in the elderly woman. *The New England Journal of Medicine, 327*, 1637-1642.

Chaudhuri, A. (2005). Why we should offer routine vitamin D supplementation in pregnancy and childhood to prevent multiple sclerosis. *Medical Hypothesis, 64*, 608-618.

Cheng, J. B., Motola, D. L., Mangelsdorf, D. J., & Russell, D. W. (2003). De-orphanization of cytochrome P450 2R1: a microsomal vitamin D 25-hydroxilase. *The Journal of Biological Chemistry, 278*(39), 38084-38093.

Chesney, R. W., & Hedberg, G. (2009). Rickets in lion cubs at the London Zoo in 1889: Some new insights. *Pediatrics, 123*(5), e948-950.

Chick, D. H. (1976). Study of rickets in Vienna 1919-1922. *Medical History, 20*(1), 41-51.

Chiu, K., Chu, A., Go, V., & Soad, M. (2004). Hypovitaminosis D is associated with insulin resistance and beta cell dysfunction. *The American Journal of Clinical Nutrition, 79*, 820-825.

Clemens, T. L., Henderson, S. L., Adams, J. S., & Holick, M. F. (1982). Increased skin pigment reduces the capacity of skin to synthesize vitamin D_3. *Lancet, 9*, 74-76.

Cockburn, F., Belton, N. R., Purvis, R. J., Giles, M. M., Brown, J. K., Turner, T. L., et al. (1980). Maternal vitamin D intake and mineral metabolism in mothers and their newborn infants. *British Medical Journal, 5*, 11-14.

Coleman, E. (1965). Infantile hypercalcaemia and cardiovascular lesions. *Archives of Disease in Childhood, 40*, 535-540.

Colston, K., Colston, M. J., & Feldman, D. (1981). 1,25-dihydroxyvitamin D_3 and malignant melanoma: the presence of receptors and inhibition of cell growth in culture. *Endocrinology, 108*(3), 1083-1086.

Cooke, R. E., & David, E. V. (1985). Serum vitamin D binding protein is a third member of the albumin and a-fetoprotein family. *The Journal of Clinical Investigation, 76*, 2420.

Council on Scientific Affairs. (1987). Vitamin preparations as dietary supplements and as therapeutic agents. *JAMA, 257*(14), 1929-1936.

Creery, R. (1953). Idiopathic hypercalcemia of infants. *Lancet, 2*, 17-23.

Crowfoot-Hodgkin, D., Webster, M., & Dunitz, J. (1957). Structure of calciferol. *Chemistry and Industry*, 1148-1149.

Cui, X., McGrath, J. J., Burne, T. H. J., Mackay-Sim, A., & Eyles, D. W. (2007). Maternal vitamin D depletion alters neurogenesis in the developing rat brain. *International Journal of Developmental Neuroscience, 25*(4), 227-232.

Cutolo, M., Otsa, K., Uprus, M., Paolino, S., & Seriolo, B. (2007). Vitamin D in rheumatoid arthritis. *Autoimmunity Reviews, 7*, 59 - 64.

Daaboul, J., Sanderson, S., Kristensen, K., & Kitson, H. (1997). Vitamin D deficiency in pregnant and breast-feeding women and their infants. *Journal of Perinatology, 17*(1), 10-14.

Daeschner, G., & Daeschner, C. (1957). Severe idiopathic hypercalcemia of infancy. *Pediatrics, 19*(3), 362-371.

Datta, S., Alfaham, M., Davies, D., Winston, J., Woodlead, S., Evans, J., et al. (2002). Vitamin D deficiency in pregnant women from a non-European ethnic minority population - an international study. *British Journal of Obstetrics and Gynaecology, 109*, 905-908.

Davies, J. (2009). A practical approach to problems of hypercalcaemia. In S. Allgrove J, NJ (Ed.): *Endocrine development calcium and bone disorders in children and adolescents*. (Vol. 16, pp. 93-114). Basel: Karger.

Davies, M., Hayes, M. E., Yin, J. A., Berry, J. L., & Mawer, E. B. (1994). Abnormal synthesis of 1,25-dihydroxyvitamin D in patients with malignant lymphoma. *The Journal of Clinical Endocrinology and Metabolism, 78*(5), 1202-1207.

Dawodu, A., Agarwal, M., Hossain, M., Kochiyil, J., & Zayed, R. (2003). Hypovitaminosis D and vitamin D deficiency in exclusively breastfeeding infants and their mothers in summer: A justification for vitamin D supplementation of breast-feeding infants. *The Journal of Pediatrics, 142*, 169-173.

Dawodu, A., Agarwal, M., Sankarankutty, M., Hardy, D., Kochiyil, J., & Badrinath, P. (2005). Higher prevalence of vitamin D deficiency in mothers of rachitic than nonrachitic children. *The Journal of Pediatrics, 147*(1), 109-111.

Dawodu, A., & Tsang, R. (2007). Vitamin D deficiency and rickets: possible role of maternal vitamin D deficiency. *Annals of Tropical Paediatrics, 27*(4), 319.

Dawodu, A., & Wagner, C. L. (2007). Mother-child vitamin D deficiency: an international perspective. *Archives of Diseases in Childhood, 92*(9), 737-740.

Dawson-Hughes, B., Heaney, R., Holick, M., Lips, P., Meunier, P., & Vieth, R. (2005). Estimates of vitamin D status. *Osteoporosis International, 16*, 713-716.

Dawson-Hughes, B., Heaney, R. P., Holick, M. F., Lips, P., Meunier, P. J., & Vieth, R. (2004). Vitamin D round table. In B. Dawson-Hughes, R. Heaney, & P. Burckhardt (Eds.), *Nutritional Aspects of Osteoporosis*. (2nd ed., pp. 263-270). Elsevier Science.

Debre, R. (1948). Toxic effects of vitamin D_2 in children. *American Journal of Diseases of Children, 75*(6), 787-791.

DeLuca, H. (1988). The vitamin D story: a collaborative effort of basic science and clinical medicine. *The FASEB Journal, 2*, 224-236.

Deluca, H. F. (1981). Recent advances in the metabolism of vitamin D. *Annual Review of Physiology, 43*, 199-209.

Delvin, E., Arabian, A., & Glorieux, F. (1978). Kinetics of liver microsomal cholecalciferol 25-hydroxylase in vitamin D-depleted and -repleted rats. *The Biochemical Journal, 172*(3), 417-422.

Delvin, E. E., Salle, B. L., Glorieux, F. H., Adeleine, P., & David, L. S. (1986). Vitamin D supplementation during pregnancy: effect on neonatal calcium homeostasis. *The Journal of Pediatrics, 109*(2), 328-334.

DeWind, L. (1961). Hypervitaminosis D with osteosclerosis. *Archives of Disease in Childhood, 36*(188), 373-380.

Dick, I., Retallack, R., & Prince, R. (1990). Rapid nongenomic inhibition of renal 25-hydroxyvitamin D_3 1-hydroxylase by 1,25-dihydroxyvitamin D_3. *The American Journal of Physiology, 259*(2 Pt 1), E272-277.

Dietrich, T., Joshipura, K. J., Dawson-Hughes, B., & Bischoff-Ferrari, H. A. (2004). Association between serum concentrations of 25-hydroxyvitamin D_3 and periodontal disease in the US population. *The American Journal of Clinical Nutrition, 80*(1), 108-113.

Dietrich, T., Nunn, M., Dawson-Hughes, B., & Bischoff-Ferrari, H. A. (2005). Association between serum concentrations of 25-hydroxyvitamin D and gingival inflammation. *The American Journal of Clinical Nutrition, 82*, 575-580.

Dowling, G., Gauvain, S., & Macrae, D. (1948). Vitamin D in the treatment of cutaneous tuberculosis. *British Medical Journal, March 6*, 430-436.

Down, P., Polak, A., & Regan, R. (1979). A family with massive acute vitamin D intoxication. *Postgraduate Medical Journal, 55*, 897-902.

Drummond, J. C., Gray, C. H., & Richardson, N. E. G. (1939). The antirachitic value of human milk. *British Medical Journal, 2*, 757-762.

Dunn, P. (1999). Professor Armand Trousseau (1801-67) and the treatment of rickets. *Archives of Disease in Childhood. Fetal and Neonatal Edition, 80*, F155-F157.

Egan, K. M., Signorello, L. B., Munro, H. M., Hargreaves, M. K., Hollis, B. W., & Blot, W. J. (2008). Vitamin D insufficiency among African-Americans in the southeastern United States: implications for cancer disparities (United States). *Cancer Causes & Control, 19*(5), 527-535.

Eisman, J., Shepard, R., & Deluca, H. (1977). Determination of 25-hydroxyvitamin D_3 in human plasma using high pressure liquid chromatography. *Analytical Biochemistry, 80*(298-305).

Eisman, J. A., Suva, L. J., Sher, E., Pearce, P. J., Funder, J. W., & Martin, T. J. (1981). Frequency of 1,25-dihydroxyvitamin D_3 receptor in human breast cancer. *Cancer Research, 41*(12 Pt 1), 5121-5124.

Elidrissy, A. T. H., Sedrani, S. H., & Lawson, D. E. M. (1984). Vitamin D deficiency in mothers of rachitic infants. *Calcified Tissue International, 36*, 266-268.

Esvelt, R. P., & De Luca, H. F. (1981). Calcitroic acid: biological activity and tissue distribution studies. *Archives of Biochemistry and Biophysics, 206*(2), 403-413.

Esvelt, R. P., Schnoes, H. K., & Deluca, H. F. (1978). Vitamin D_3 from rat skins irradiated *in vitro* with ultraviolet light. *Archives of Biochemistry and Biophysics, 188*, 282-286.

Eugster, E. A., Sane, K. S., & Brown, D. M. (1996). Need for a policy change to support vitamin D supplementation. *Minnesota Medicine, 79*, 29-32.

Evans, R. M. (1988). The steroid and thyroid hormone receptor superfamily. *Science, 240*(4854), 889-95.

Eyles, D., Brown, J., MacKay-Sim, A., McGrath, J., & Feron, F. (2003). Vitamin D_3 and brain development. *Neuroscience, 118*(3), 641-653.

Eyles, D., Smith, S., Kinobeb, R., Hewison, M., & McGrath, J. (2005). Distribution of the vitamin D receptor and 1a-hydroxylase in human brain. *Journal of Chemical Neuroanatomy, 29*, 21-30.

Fanconi, G., Giradet, P., Schlesinger, B., Butler, N., & Black, J. (1952). Chronische hypercalcamie, kombiniert mit osteosklerose, hyperazotamie, minderwuchs und kongenitalen missbildungen. *Helvetica Paediatrica Acta, 7*, 314.

Favus, M. (1999). Laboratory values of importance for calcium metabolic bone disease. In M. Favus (Ed.), *Primer on the metabolic bone diseases and disorders of mineral metabolism* (4th ed., pp. 467-470). New York: Lippincott, Williams & Wilkins.

Favus, M., & Long, C. (1986). Evidence for calcium-dependent control of 1,25-dihydroxyvitamin D_3 production by rat kidney proximal tubules. *The Journal of Biological Chemistry, 261*, 11224-11229.

Feldman, D., Krishnan, A., Moreno, J., Swami, S., Peehl, D. M., & Srinivas, S. (2007). Vitamin D inhibition of the prostaglandin pathway as therapy for prostate cancer. *Nutrition Reviews, 65*(8 Pt 2), S113-115.

Feron, F., Burne, T., Brown, J., Smith, E., McGrath, J., Mackay-Sim, A., et al. (2005). Developmental vitamin D-3 deficiency alters the adult rat brain. *Brain Research Bulletin, 65*, 141-148.

Fischer, E. I. C., Armentano, R. L., Levenson, J., Barra, G., Morales, M. C., Breitbart, G. J., et al. (1991). Paradoxically decreased aortic wall stiffness in response to vitamin D_3-induced calcinosis. *Circulation Research, 68*, 1549-1559.

Food and Nutrition Board. Standing Committee on the Scientific Evaluation of Dietary Reference Intakes. (1997). *Dietary reference intakes for calcium, phosphorus, magnesium, vitamin D, and fluoride.* Washington, D.C.: National Academy Press.

Ford, E. S., Ajani, U. A., McGuire, L. C., & Liu, S. (2005). Concentrations of serum vitamin D and the metabolic syndrome among U.S. adults. *Diabetes Care, 28*(5), 1228-1230.

Forman, J. P., Giovannucci, E., Holmes, M. D., Bischoff-Ferrari, H. A., Tworoger, S. S., Willett, W. C., et al. (2007). Plasma 25-hydroxyvitamin D levels and risk of incident hypertension. *Hypertension, 49*(5), 1063-1069.

Fox, J., Kollenkirchen, U., & Walters, M. (1991). Deficiency of vitamin D metabolites directly stimulates renal 25-hydroxyvitamin D_3-1-hydroxylase activity in rats. *Metabolism, 40*(4), 438-441.

Fraser, D. R. (1980). Regulation of the metabolism of vitamin D. *Physiological Reviews, 60*(2), 551-613.

Fraser, D. R. (1983). The physiological economy of vitamin D. *Lancet, 1*(8331), 969-972.

Fraser, D. R., & Kodicek, E. (1970). Unique biosynthesis by kidney of a biological active vitamin D metabolite. *Nature, 228*(5273), 764-766.

Freedman, D. M., Chang, S. C., Falk, R. T., Purdue, M. P., Huang, W. Y., McCarty, C. A., et al. (2008). Serum levels of vitamin D metabolites and breast cancer risk in the prostate, lung, colorectal, and ovarian cancer screening trial. *Cancer Epidemiology, Biomarkers, & Prevention, 17*(4), 889-894.

Friedman, W. F. (1967). Vitamin D as a cause of the supravalvular aortic stenosis syndrome. *American Heart Journal, 73*, 718-720.

Friedman, W. F., & Mills, L. (1969). The relationship between vitamin D and the craniofacial and dental anomalies of the supravalvular aortic stenosis syndrome. *Pediatrics, 43*, 12-18.

Friedman, W. F., & Mills, L. S. (1967). The production of "elfin facies" and abnormal dentition by vitamin D during pregnancy: relationship to the supravalvular aortic stenosis syndrome. *Proc. Soc. Pediatr. Res., 37*, 80.

Friedman, W. F., & Roberts, W. C. (1966). Vitamin D and the supravalvular aortic stenosis syndrome. The transplacental effects of vitamin D on the aorta of the rabbit. *Circulation, 34*, 77-86.

Fuleihan, G.-H., Nabulsi, M., Choucair, M., Salamoun, M., Shahine, C., Kizirian, A., et al. (2001). Hypovitaminosis D in Healthy Schoolchildren. *Pediatrics, 107*(4), e53-e57.

Fuleihan, G. E., & Deeb, M. (1999). Hypovitaminosis D in a sunny country. *The New England Journal of Medicine, 340*(23), 1840-1841.

Garabedian, M., Holick, M., Deluca, H., & Boyle, I. (1972). Control of 25-Hydroxycholecalciferol Metabolism by Parathyroid Glands. *Proceedings of the National Academy of Sciences of the United States of America, 69, 1673-1676.*

Garabedian, M., Pavlovitch, H., Fellot, C., & Balsan, S. (1974). Metabolism of 25-hydroxyvitamin D_3 in anephric rats: a new active metabolite. *Proceedings of the National Academy of Sciences of the United States of America, 71*(2), 554-557.

Garabedian, M., Tanaka, Y., Holick, M. F., & Deluca, H. F. (1974). Response of intestinal calcium transport and bone calcium mobilization to 1,25-dihydroxyvitamin D_3 in thyroparathyroidectomized rats. *Endocrinology, 94*(4), 1022-1027.

Garcia, R. E., Friedman, W. F., Kaback, M., & Rowe, R. D. (1964). Idiopathic hypercalcemia and supravalvular aortic stenosis: Documentation of a new syndrome. *The New England Journal of Medicine, 271*, 117-120.

Garland, C., Comstock, G., Garland, F., Helsing, K., Shaw, E., & Gorham, E. (1989). Serum 25(OH) D and colon cancer: Eight-year prospective study. *Lancet, 2*, 1176-1178.

Garland, C., Gorham, E., Mohr, S., Grant, W., Giovannucci, E., & Lipkin, M. (2007). Vitamin D and prevention of breast. cancer: Pooled analysis. *Journal of Steroids and Biochemistry, 103*, 708-711.

Garland, F., Garland, C., Gorham, E., & Young, J. (1990). Geographic variation in breast cancer mortality in the United States: A hypothesis involving exposure to solar radiation. *Preventive Medicine, 19*, 614-622.

Gartner, L. M., Greer, F. R., American Academy of Pediatrics, Section on Breastfeeding & Committee on Nutrition. (2003). Prevention of Rickets and Vitamin D Deficiency: New Guidelines for Vitamin D Intake. *Pediatrics, 111*(4), 908-910.

Gessner, B. D., deSchweinitz, E., Petersen, K. M., & Lewandowski, C. (1997). Nutritional rickets among breast-fed black and Alaska Native children. *Alaska Medicine, 39*(3), 72-74, 87.

Gessner, B. D., Plotnik, J., & Muth, P. T. (2003). 25-hydroxyvitamin D levels among healthy children in Alaska. *The Journal of Pediatrics, 143*(4), 434-437.

Ghazarian, J. G. (1990). The renal mitochondrial hydroxylases of the vitamin D_3 endocrine complex: how are they regulated at the molecular level. *Journal of Bone and Mineral Research, 5*(9), 897-903.

Ghazarian, J. G., Jefcoate, C. R., Knutson, J. C., Orme-Johnson, W. H., & Deluca, H. F. (1974). Mitochondrial cytochrome P_{450}: A component of chick kidney 25(OH)D-1a-hydroxylase. *The Journal of Biological Chemistry, 249*, 3026-3033.

Giovannucci, E. (2005). The epidemiology of vitamin D and cancer incidence and mortality: A review (United States). *Cancer Causes & Control, 16*, 83-95.

Giovannucci, E. (2007). Strengths and limitations of current epidemiologic studies: vitamin D as a modifier of colon and prostate cancer risk. *Nutrition Reviews, 65*(8 Pt 2), S77-79.

Giovannucci, E., Liu, Y., Hollis, B. W., & Rimm, E. B. (2008). 25-Hydroxyvitamin D and Risk of Myocardial Infarction in Men: A Prospective Study. *Archives of Internal Medicine, 168*(11), 1174-1180.

Giovannucci, E., Liu, Y., Rimm, E. B., Hollis, B. W., Fuchs, C. S., Stampfer, M. J., et al. (2006). Prospective study of predictors of vitamin D status and cancer incidence and mortality in men. *Journal of the National Cancer Institute, 98*(7), 451-459.

Glissen, F. (1668). *A treatise of the rickets being a disease common to children.* London.

Glissen, F. (1650). *De Rachitide sive morbo puerili, qui vulgo The Rickets diciteur.* London.

Gloth, F. M., Gundberg, C. M., Hollis, B. W., Haddad, J. G., & Tobin, J. D. (1995). Vitamin D deficiency in homebound elderly persons. *JAMA, 274*, 1683-1686.

Gloth, F. M., Tobin, J. D., Sherman, S. S., & Hollis, B. W. (1991). Is the recommended daily allowance for vitamin D too low for the homebound elderly? *The Journal of the American Society for Geriatric Dentistry, 39*, 137-141.

Goff, J. P., Horst, R. L., & Littledike, E. (1984). Effect of low vitamin D status at parturition on the vitamin D status of neonatal piglets. *The Journal of Nutrition, 114*, 163-169.

Goldblatt, H., & Soames, K. (1923). A study of rats on a normal diet irradiated daily by the mercury vapor quartz lamp or kept in darkness. *The Biochemical Journal, 17*, 294-297.

Goodenday, L. S., & Gordon, G. S. (1971). No risk from vitamin D in pregnancy. *Annals of Internal Medicine, 75*, 807.

Gordon, C. M., Williams, A. L., Feldman, H. A., May, J., Sinclair, L., Vasquez, A., et al. (2008). Treatment of hypovitaminosis D in infants and toddlers. *The Journal of Clinical Endocrinology and Metabolism, 93*(7), 2716-2721.

Grant, W. B. (2002). An estimate of premature cancer mortality in the US due to inadequate doses of solar ultraviolet-B radiation. *Cancer, 94*, 1867-1875.

Gray, R. (1987). Evidence that somatomedins mediate the effect of hypophosphatemia to increase serum 1,25-dihydroxyvitamin D_3 levels in rats. *Endocrinology, 121*(2), 504-512.

Gray, R., Garthwaite, T., & Phillips, L. (1983). Growth hormone and triiodothyronine permit an increase in plasma 1,25(OH)2D concentrations in response to dietary phosphate deprivation in hypophysectomized rats. *Calcified Tissue International, 35*(1), 100-106.

Gray, T. K., Lester, G. E., & Lorenc, R. S. (1979). Evidence for extra-renal 1 alpha-hydroxylation of 25-hydroxyvitamin D_3 in pregnancy. *Science, 204*(4399), 1311-1313.

Greer, F. R. (2004). Issues in establishing vitamin D recommendations for infants and children. *The American Journal of Clinical Nutrition, 80*(6), 1759S-1762.

Greer, F. R., Hollis, B. W., Cripps, D. J., & Tsang, R. C. (1984). Effects of maternal ultraviolet B irradiation on vitamin D content of human milk. *Journal of Pediatrics, 105*, 431-433.

Greer, F. R., Hollis, B. W., & Napoli, J. L. (1984). High concentrations of vitamin D_2 in human milk associated with pharmacologic doses of vitamin D_2. *Journal of Pediatrics, 105*, 61-64.

Greer, F. R., & Marshall, S. (1989). Bone mineral content, serum vitamin D metabolite concentrations and ultraviolet B light exposure in infants fed human milk with and without vitamin D_2 supplements. *Journal of Pediatrics, 114*, 204-212.

Grosse, B., Bourdeau, A., & Lieberherr, M. (1993). Oscillations in inositol 1,4,5-trisphosphate and diacyglycerol induced by vitamin D_3 metabolites in confluent mouse osteoblasts. *Journal of Bone and Mineral Research, 8*(9), 1059-1069.

Guo, Y. D., Strugnell, S., Back, D. W., & Jones, G. (1993). Transfected human liver cytochrome P-450 hydroxylates vitamin D analogs at different side-chain positions. *Proceedings of the National Academy of Sciences in the United States of America, 90*(18), 8668-8672.

Guoth, M., Murgia, A., Smith, R. M., & et.al. (1990). Cell surface vitamin D-binding protein is acquired from plasma. *Endocrinology, 125*, 2313.

Guy, R. (1923). The history of cod liver oil as a remedy. *American Journal of Diseases of Children, 26*, 112-116.

Haddad, J. G. (1992). Clinical aspects of measurement of vitamin D sterols and the vitamin D binding protein. In F. L. Coe & M. J. Vavus (Eds.), *Disorder of Bone and Mineral Metabolism* (pp. 195-216). New York: Raven.

Haddad, J. G., & Chyu, K. (1971). Competitive protein-binding radioassay for 25-hydroxycholecalciferol. *The Journal of Clinical Endocrinology and Metabolism, 33*, 992-995.

Haddad, J. G., Jr., & Hahn, T. J. (1973). Natural and synthetic sources of circulating 25-hydroxyvitamin D in man. *Nature, 244*(5417), 515-517.

Haddad, J. G., & Kyung, J. C. (1971). Competitive protein-binding radioassay for 25(OH)D_3. *The Journal of Clinical Endocrinology and Metabolism, 33*, 992-995.

Haddad, J. G., Matsuoka, L. Y., Hollis, B. W., Hu, Y., & Wortsman, J. (1993). Human plasma transport of vitamin D after its endogenous synthesis. *The Journal of Clinical Investigation, 91*(6), 2552-2555.

Haddad, J. G., & Stamp, T. C. B. (1974). Circulating 25-hydroxyvitamin D in man. *The American Journal of Medicine, 57*, 57-62.

Haddock, L., Corcino, J., & Vazquez, M. D. (1982). 25(OH)D serum levels in the normal Puerto Rican population and in subjects with tropical sprue and parathyroid disease. *Puerto Rico Health Sciences Journal, 1*, 85-91.

Hahn, T. J., & Halstead, L. R. (1979). Anticonvulsant drug-induced osteomalacia: alterations in mineral metabolism and response to vitamin D_3 administration. *Calcified Tissue International, 27*(1), 13-18.

Ham, A., & Lewis, M. (1934). Hypervitaminosis D rickets: The action of vitamin D. *British Journal of Experimental Pathology, 15*, 228-234.

Harkness, L., & Cromer, B. (2005a). Low levels of 25-hydroxy vitamin D are associated with elevated parathyroid hormone in healthy adolescent females. *Osteoporosis International, 16*(1), 109-113.

Harkness, L. S., & Cromer, B. A. (2005b). Vitamin D deficiency in adolescent females. *The Journal of Adolescent Health, 37*(1), 75.

Harris, B. S., & Bunket, J. W. M. (1939). Vitamin D potency of human breast milk. *American Journal of Public Health, 29*, 744-747.

Harris, L., & Innes, J. (1931). XLV. The mode of action of vitamin D. Studies on hypervitaminosis D. The influence of the calcium-phosphate intake. *The Biochemical Journal, 25*, 367-390.

Harris, L., & Moore, T. (1928). CCXXXII. "Hypervitaminosis" and "vitamin balance". *The Biochemical Journal, 22*, 1461-1477.

Harris, S. S. (2005). Vitamin D in type 1 diabetes prevention. *The Journal of Nutrition, 135*(2), 323-325.

Harrison, H. E. (1996). The disappearance of rickets. *American Journal of Public Health, 56*, 734-737.

Hathcock, J. N., Shao, A., Vieth, R., & Heaney, R. (2007). Risk assessment for vitamin D. *The American Journal of Clinical Nutrition, 85*(1), 6-18.

Hatun, S., Ozkan, B., Orbak, Z., Doneray, H., Cizmecioglu, F., Toprak, D., et al. (2005). Vitamin D deficiency in early infancy. *The Journal of Nutrition, 135*(2), 279-282.

Hayes, C. E. (2000). Vitamin D: a natural inhibitor of multiple sclerosis. *The Proceedings of the Nutrition Society, 59*, 531-535.

Heaney, R., Dowell, M., Hale, C., & Bendich, A. (2003). Calcium absorption varies within the reference range for serum 25-hydroxyvitamin D. *Journal of the American College of Nutrition, 22*(2), 142-146.

Heaney, R. P., Davies, K. M., Chen, T. C., Holick, M. F., & Barger-Lux, M. J. (2003). Human serum 25-hydroxycholecalciferol response to extended oral dosing with cholecalciferol. *American Journal of Clinical Nutrition, 77*, 204-210.

Hess, A. (1922). Infantile rickets: the significance of clinical, radiographic, and chemical explanations in its diagnosis and incidence. *American Journal of Diseases of Children, xxiv*, 327.

Hess, A. F. (1929). The history of rickets. *In: Rickets Including Osteomalacia and Tetany.* Lea and Febiger (eds), Philadelphia, PA, 22-37.

Hess, A., & Unger, L. (1921a). The cure of infantile rickets by sunlight. *JAMA, 77*, 1,39.

Hess, A., & Unger L. (1922a). Infantile rickets: The significance of clinical, radiographic and chemical examinations in its diagnosis and incidence. *American Journal of Diseases of Children, 24,* 327-338.

Hess, A. F., &. Unger, L. J (1921b). An interpretation of the seasonal variation of rickets. *American Journal of Diseases of Children, 22,* 2, 186-192.

Hess, A. F., Unger, L. J., et al. (1922b). Experimental rickets in rats: Vii. The prevention of rickets by sunlight, by the rays of the mercury vapor lamp, and by the carbon arc lamp. *The Journal of Experimental Medicine, 36,* 4, 427-446.

Hess, A. F., Unger, L. J., et al. (1922c). "Experimental Rickets in Rats : Viii. The Effect of Roentgen Rays." *The Journal of Experimental Medicine, 36,* 4, 447-452.

Hess, A. F. & Weinstock, M. (1923). "A study of light waves in their relation to rickets." *Journal of the American Medical Association, 80,* 10, 687-690.

Heubi, J. E., Hollis, B. W., Specker, B., & Tsang, R. C. (1989). Bone disease in chronic childhood cholestasis. I. Vitamin D absorption and metabolism. *Hepatology, 9*(2), 258-264.

Heubi, J. E., Hollis, B. W., & Tsang, R. C. (1990). Bone disease in chronic childhood cholestasis. II. Better absorption of 25-OH vitamin D than vitamin D in extrahepatic biliary atresia. *Pediatric Research, 27*(1), 26-31.

Hild, J. (1942). Calcification of arteries and deposits of calcium in both lungs in an infant. *American Journal of Diseases of Children, 63*, 126-130.

Hillman, L. S., & Haddad, J. G. (1974). Human perinatal vitamin D metabolism. I. 25-Hydroxyvitamin D in maternal and cord blood. *The Journal of Pediatrics, 84*(5), 742-749.

Hinek, A., & Poole, A. R. (1988). The influence of vitamin D metabolites on the calcification of cartilage matrix and the C-propeptide of type II collagen (chondrocalcin). *Journal of Bone and Mineral Research, 3*(4), 421-429.

Ho, M. L., Yen, H. C., Tsang, R. C., Specker, B. L., Chen, X. C., & Nichols, B. L. (1985). Randomized study of sunshine exposure and serum 25-OHD in breast-fed infants in Beijing, China. *The Journal of Pediatrics, 107*(6), 928-931.

Holick, M. F. (1992). Evolutionary biology and pathology of vitamin D. *Journal of Nutritional Science and Vitaminology (Tokyo), Spec No*, 79-83.

Holick, M. F. (1994). McCollum Award Lecture, 1994: Vitamin D--new horizons for the 21st century. *The American Journal of Clinical Nutrition, 60*(4), 619-630.

Holick, M. F. (1995a). Environmental factors that influence the cutaneous production of vitamin D. *The American Journal of Clinical Nutrition, 61*, 638S-645S.

Holick, M. F. (1995b). Noncalcemic actions of 1,25-dihydroxyvitamin D_3 and clinical applications. *Bone, 17*(2, Supplement), 107S-111S.

Holick, M. F. (2004). Vitamin D: Importance in the prevention of cancers, type 1 diabetes, heart disease, and osteoporosis. *The Americn Journal of Clinical Nutrition, 79*, 362-371.

Holick, M. F. (2007a). Vitamin D deficiency. *The New England Journal of Medicine, 357*(3), 266-281.

Holick, M. F. (2007b). Optimal vitamin D status for the prevention and treatment of osteoporosis. *Drugs & Aging, 24*, 1017-1029.

Holick, M. F., Biancuzzo, R. M., Chen, T. C., Klein, E. K., Young, A., Bibuld, D., et al. (2008). Vitamin D_2 is as effective as Vitamin D_3 in maintaining circulating concentrations of 25-hydroxyvitamin D. *The Journal of Clinical Endocrinology and Metabolism, 93*(3), 677-681.

Holick, M. F., & Clark, M. B. (1978). The photobiogenesis and metabolism of vitamin D. *Federation Proceedings, 37*(12), 2567-2574.

Holick, M. F., MacLaughlin, J. A., Clark, M. B., Holick, S. A., Pitts, J. T., Anderson, R. R., et al. (1980). Photosynthesis of vitamin D_3 in human skin and its physiologic consequences. *Science, 210*, 203-205.

Holick, M. F., MacLaughlin, J. A., & Doppelt, S. H. (1981a). Factors that influence the cutaneous photosynthesis of previtamin D_3. *Science, 211*, 590-593.

Holick, M. F., MacLaughlin, J. A., & Doppelt, S. H. (1981b). Regulation of cutaneous previtamin D_3 photosynthesis in man: skin pigment is not an essential regulator. *Science, 211*(4482), 590-593.

Holick, M. F., Perez, A., & Raab, R.. (1992). 1,25-Dihydroxyvitamin D_3 for the treatment of psoriasis. *Journal of Nutritional Science and Vitaminology (Tokyo) Spec No*: 84-87.

Holick, M. F., Schnoes, H. K., & DeLuca, H. F. (1971). Identification of 1,25-dihydroxycholecalciferol, a form of vitamin D_3 metabolically active in the intestine. *Proceedings of the National Academy of Sciences of the United States of America, 68*(4), 803-804.

Holick, M. F., Schnoes, H. K., DeLuca, H. F., Suda, T., & Cousins, R. J. (1971). Isolation and identification of 1,25-dihydroxycholecalciferol. A metabolite of vitamin D active in intestine. *Biochemistry, 10*(14), 2799-2804.

Holick, M. F., Shao, Q., Liu, W. W., & Chen, T. C. (1992). The vitamin D content of fortified milk and infant formula. *The New England Journal of Medicine, 326*(18), 1178-1181.

Hollander, D., Muralidhara, K., & Zimmerman, A. (1978). Vitamin D$_3$ intestinal absorption *in vivo*: influence of fatty acids, bile salts, and perfusate pH on absorption. *Gut, 19*, 267-272

Hollis, B. W. (1983). Individual quantitation of vitamin D$_2$, vitamin D$_3$, 25(OH)D$_2$ and 25(OH)D$_3$ in human milk. *Analytical Biochemistry, 131*, 211-219.

Hollis, B. W. (1984). Comparison of equilibrium and disequilibrium assay conditions for ergocalceferol, cholecaliferol and their major metabolites. *Journal of Steroid Biochemistry*, 81-86.

Hollis, B. W. (1986). Assay of circulating 1,25-dihydroxyvitamin D involving a novel single cartridge extraction and purification procedure. *Clinical Chemistry, 32*, 11, 2060-2063.

Hollis, B. W. (1990). 25-Hydroxyvitamin D$_3$-1 alpha-hydroxylase in porcine hepatic tissue: subcellular localization to both mitochondria and microsomes. *Proceedings of the National Academy of Sciences in the United States of America, 87*(16), 6009-6013.

Hollis, B. W. (1996). Assessment of vitamin D nutritional and hormonal status: What to measure and how to do it. *Calcified Tissue International, 58*, 4-5.

Hollis, B. W. (2005). Circulating 25-hydroxyvitamin D levels indicative of vitamin d sufficiency: implications for establishing a new effective dietary intake recommendation for vitamin D. *The Journal of Nutrition, 135*(2), 317-322.

Hollis, B. W. (2007). Vitamin D requirement during pregnancy and lactation. *Journal of Bone and Mineral Research, 22*(Suppl 2), V39-V44).

Hollis, B. W. (2009). US recommendations fail to correct vitamin D deficiency. *Nature Reviews. Endocrinology, 5*, 1-2.

Hollis, B. W., & Horst, R. L. (2007). The assessment of circulating 25(OH)D and 1,25(OH)2D: where we are and where we are going. *The Journal of Steroid Biochemistry and Molecular Biology 103*, 3-5, 473-476.

Hollis, B. W., Kamerud, J. Q., Selvaag, S. R., Lorenz, J. D., & Napoli, J. L. (1993). Determination of vitamin D status by radioimmunoassay with an ^{125}I-labeled tracer. *Clinical Chemistry, 39*, 529-533.

Hollis, B. W., & Pittard, W. B. (1984). Evaluation of the total fetomaternal vitamin D relationships at term: Evidence for racial differences. *The Journal of Clinical Endocrinology and Metabolism, 59*, 652-657.

Hollis, B. W., Pittard, W. B., & Reinhardt, T. A. (1986). Relationships among vitamin D, 25(OH)D, and vitamin D-binding protein concentrations in the plasma and milk of human subjects. *The Journal of Clinical Endocrinology and Metabolism, 62*, 41-44.

Hollis, B. W., Roos, B. A., Drapper, H. H., & Lambert, P. W. (1981a). Occurrence of vitamin D sulfate in human milk whey. *The Journal of Nutrition, 111*, 2, 384-390.

Hollis, B. W., Roos, B., Draper, H. H., & Lambert, P. W. (1981b). Vitamin D and its metabolites in human and bovine milk. *The Journal of Nutrition, 111*, 1240-1248.

Hollis, B., Roos, B., & Lambert, P. (1980). 25,26-Dihydroxycholecalciferol: a precursor in the renal synthesis of 25-hydroxycholecalciferol-26,23-lactone. *Biochem Biophys Res Commun, 95*(2), 520-528.

Hollis, B. W., Roos, B. A., & Lambert, P. W. (1981). Vitamin D in plasma: Quantitation by a nonequilbrium ligand binding assay." *Steroids, 37*, 6, 609-619.

Hollis, B. W., Roos, B. A., & Lambert, P. W. (1982). Vitamin D compounds in human and bovine milk. *Advances in Nutritional Research, 4,* 59-75.

Hollis, B. W., & Wagner, C. L. (2004a). Assessment of dietary vitamin D requirements during pregnancy and lactation. *The American Journal of Clinical Nutrition, 79,* 717 - 726.

Hollis, B. W., & Wagner, C. L. (2004b). Vitamin D requirements during lactation: High-dose maternal supplementation as therapy to prevent hypovitaminosis D in both mother and nursing infant. *The American Journal of Clinical Nutrition, 80S,* 1752S-1758S.

Hollis, B. W., Wagner, C. L., Drezner, M. K., & Binkley, N. C. (2007). Circulating vitamin D_3 and 25-hydroxyvitamin D in humans: An important tool to define adequate nutritional vitamin D status. *The Journal of Steroid Biochemistry and Molecular Biology, 103*(3-5), 631-634.

Hollis, B. W., Wagner, C. L., Kratz, A., Sluss, P. M., & Lewandrowski, K. B. (2005). Normal serum vitamin D levels. Correspondence. *The New England Journal of Medicine, 352,* 515-516.

Hopkins, F. (1906). The analyst and the medical man. *Analyst, 31,* 385-404.

Horst, R. L., Reinhardt, T. A., & Reddy, G. S. (2005). Vitamin D metabolism. In D. Feldman, J. W. Pike, & F. H. Glorieux (Eds.), *Vitamin D* (p. 16). New York: Elsevier Academic Press.

Howard, G. A., Turner, R. T., Sherrard, D. J., & Baylink, D. J. (1981). Human bone cells in culture metabolize 25-hydroxyvitamin D_3 to 1,25-dihydroxyvitamin D_3 and 24,25-dihydroxyvitamin D_3. *The Journal of Biological Chemistry, 256*(15), 7738-7740.

Howard, J., & Meyer, R. (1948). Intoxication with vitamin D. *The Journal of Clinical Endocrinology, 8*(11), 895-909.

Hu, J., Morrison, H., Mery, L., DesMeules, M., Macleod, M., & Canadian Cancer Registries Epidemiology Research, G. (2007). Diet and vitamin or mineral supplementation and risk of colon cancer by subsite in Canada. *European Journal of Cancer Prevention, 16*(4), 275-291.

Hurley, D., & Singh, R. (2006). Vitamin D deficiency--A new understanding. *Endocrinology Updates, 1*(2), 4-5.

Hypponen, E. (2004). Micronutrients and the risk of type 1 diabetes: vitamin D, vitamin E, and nicotinamide. *Nutrition Reviews, 62*(9), 340-347.

Hypponen, E. (2005). Vitamin D for the prevention of preeclampsia? A hypothesis. *Nutrition Reviews, 63*(7), 225-232.

Hypponen, E., Hartikainen, A. L., Sovio, U., Jarvelin, M. R., & Pouta, A. (2007). Does vitamin D supplementation in infancy reduce the risk of pre-eclampsia? *European Journal of Clinical Nutrition, 61*(9), 1136-1139.

Hypponen, E., Laara, E., Reunanen, A., Jarvelin, M. R., & Virtanen, S. M. (2001). Intake of vitamin D and risk of type 1 diabetes: A birth-cohort study. *Lancet, 358,* 1500-1503.

Hypponen, E., & Power, C. (2007). Hypovitaminosis D in British adults at age 45 y: nationwide cohort study of dietary and lifestyle predictors. *The American Journal of Clinical Nutrition, 85,* 860 - 868.

Hypponen, E., Sovio, U., Wjst, M., Patel, S., Pekkanen, J., Hartikainen, A. L., et al. (2004). Infant vitamin D supplementation and allergic conditions in adulthood: northern Finland birth cohort 1966. *Annals of the New York Academy of Sciences, 1037*, 84-95.

Ingles, S. A. (2007). Can diet and/or sunlight modify the relationship between vitamin D receptor polymorphisms and prostate cancer risk? *Nutr Rev, 65*(8 Pt 2), S105-107.

Institute of Medicine. (1990a). Calcium, Vitamin D, and Magnesium. *Subcommittee on Nutritional Status and Weight Gain during Pregnancy: Nutrition During Pregnancy* (pp. 318-335). Washington, D.C.: National Academy Press.

Institute of Medicine. (1990b). *Nutrition During Lactation*. Washington, D.C.: National Academy Press.

Jacobs, E. T., Alberts, D. S., Foote, J. A., Green, S. B., Hollis, B. W., Yu, Z., et al. (2008). Vitamin D insufficiency in southern Arizona. *The American Journal of Clinical Nutrition, 87*(3), 608-613.

Jacobus, C. H., Holick, M. F., Shao, Q., Chen, T. C., Holm, I. A., Kolodny, J. M., et al. (1992). Hypervitaminosis D associated with drinking milk. *The New England Journal of Medicine, 326*(18), 1173-1177.

Javaid, M. K., Crozier, S. R., Harvey, N. C., Gale, C. R., Dennison, E. M., Boucher, B. J., et al. (2006). Maternal vitamin D status during pregnancy and childhood bone mass at age 9 years: a longitudinal study. *The Lancet, 367*(9504), 36-43.

Jeans, P., & Stearns, G. (1938). The effect of vitamin D on linear growth in infancy. II. The effect of intakes above 1,800 U.S.P. units daily. *The Journal of Pediatrics, 13*, 730-740.

Johnson, D., C. Wagner, et al. (2010). Vitamin D deficiency is common in pregnancy. *American Journal of Perinatology, in press.*

Kamen, D. L., Cooper, G. S., Bouali, H., Shaftman, S. R., Hollis, B. W., & Gilkeson, G. S. (2006). Vitamin D deficiency in systemic lupus erythematosus. *Autoimmunity Reviews, 5*(2), 114-117.

Kawashima, H., & Kurokawa, K. (1982). Localization of receptors for 1,25-dihydroxyvitamin D, along the rat nephron. Direct evidence for presence of the receptors in both proximal and distal nephron. *The Journal of Biological Chemistry, 257*(22), 13428-13432.

Kawashima, H., Torikai, S., & Kurokawa, K. (1981a). Calcitonin selectively stimulates 25-hydroxyvitamin D$_3$-1 alpha-hydroxylase in proximal straight tubule of rat kidney. *Nature, 291*(5813), 327-329.

Kawashima, H., Torikai, S., & Kurokawa, K. (1981b). Localization of 25-hydroxyvitamin D$_3$ 1 alpha-hydroxylase and 24-hydroxylase along the rat nephron. *Proceedings of the National Academy of Sciences of the United States of America, 78*(2), 1199-1203.

Kesby, J., Burne, T., McGrath, J., & Eyles, D. (2006). Developmental vitamin D deficiency alters MK 801-induced hyperlocomotion in the adult rat: an animal model of schizophrenia. *Biological Psychiatry, 60*, 591-596.

Kieseier, B., Giovannoni, G., & Hartung, H. (1999). Immunological surrogate markers of disease activity in multiple sclerosis. *Electroencephalography and Clinical Neurophysiology. Supplement, 50*, 570 - 583.

Kimball, S. M., Ursell, M. R., O'Connor, P., & Vieth, R. (2007). Safety of vitamin D$_3$ in adults with multiple sclerosis. *The American Journal of Clinical Nutrition, 86*(3), 645-651.

Kleinman, R. (Ed.). (2009). *Pediatric nutrition handbook* (6th ed.). Elk Grove Village, IL: American Academy of Pediatrics.

Knudtzon, J., Aksnes, L., Akslen, L. A., & Aarskog, D. (1987). Elevated 1,25-dihydroxyvitamin D and normocalcaemia in presumed familial Williams Syndrome. *Clinical Genetics, 32*, 369-374.

Ko, P., Burkert, R., McGrath, J., & Eyles, D. (2004). Maternal vitamin D$_3$ deprivation and the regulation of apoptosis and cell cyle during rat brain development. *Developmental Brain Research, 153*, 61-68.

Kovacs, C. S. (2008). Vitamin D in pregnancy and lactation: maternal, fetal, and neonatal outcomes from human and animal studies. *The American Journal of Clinical Nutrition, 88*(2), 520S-528.

Krall, E. A., Wehler, C., Garcia, R. I., Harris, S. S., & Dawson-Hughes, B. (2001). Calcium and vitamin D supplements reduce tooth loss in the elderly. *The American Journal of Medicine, 111*(6), 452-456.

Kramer, B., H. Casparis, et al. (1922). Ultraviolet radiation in rickets: Effect on the calcium and inorganic phosphorus concentration of the serum. *American Journal of Diseases of Children 24*, 1, 20-26.

Kreiter, S. (2001). The reemergence of vitamin D deficiency rickets-the need for vitamin D supplementation. In: *AMB News and Views. The Newsletter of the Academy of Breastfeeding Medicine,* p. 1 and 5.

Kreiter, S. R., Schwartz, R. P., Kirkman, H. N., Charlton, P. A., Calikoglu, A. S., & Davenport, M. L. (2000). Nutritional rickets in African American breast-fed infants. *The Journal of Pediatrics, 137*(2), 153-157.

Kreitmair, & Moll, H. A. (1928). *Munch med Woch, 15*, 637.

Kumar, R., Nagubandi, S., & Londowski, J. M. (1980). The enterohepatic physiology of 24,25-dihydroxyvitamin D$_3$. *The Journal of Laboratory and Clinical Medicine, 96*(2), 278-284.

Kumar, R., Nagubandi, S., Mattox, V. R., & Londowski, J. M. (1980). Enterohepatic physiology of 1,25-dihydroxyvitamin D$_3$. *The Journal of Clinical Investigation, 65*(2), 277-284.

Kussmann, M., & Affolter, M. (2009). Proteomics at the center of nutrigenomics: Comprehensive molecular understanding of dietary health effects. *Nutrition, 25*(11-12), 1085-1093.

Laaksi, I., Ruohola, J. P., Tuohimaa, P., Auvinen, Al, Haataja, R., Pihlajamaki, H., Ylikomi, T. (2007). An association of serum vitamin D concentrations < 40 nmol/L with acute respiratory tract infection in young Finnish men. *The American Journal of Clinical Nutrition 86*, 3, 714-717.

Labuda, M., Lemieux, N., Tihy, F., Prinster, C., & Glorieux, F. H. (1993). Human 25-hydroxyvitamin D 24-hydroxylase cytochrome P450 subunit maps to a different chromosomal location than that of pseudovitamin D-deficient rickets. *Journal of Bone and Mineral and Research, 8*(11), 1397-1406.

Ladhani, S., Srinivasan, L., Buchanan, C., & Allgrove, J. (2004). Presentation of vitamin D deficiency. *Archives of Disease in Childhood, 89*, 781-784.

Ladizesky, M., Lu, Z., Oliveri, B., San Roman, N., Diaz, S., Holick, M. F., et al. (1995). Solar ultraviolet B radiation and photoproduction of vitamin D$_3$ in central and southern areas of Argentina. *Journal of Bone and Mineral Research, 10*(4), 545-549.

Lagunova, Z., Porojnicu, A. C., Lindberg, F., Hexeberg, S., & Moan, J. (2009). The dependency of vitamin D status on body mass index, gender, age and season. *Anticancer Research, 29*(9), 3713-3720.

Lakdawala, D. R., & Widdowson, E. M. (1977). Vitamin D in human milk. *Lancet, 1*, 167-168.

Lambert, P. W., Stern, P. H., Avioli, R. C., Brackett, N. C., Turner, R. T., Greene, A., et al. (1982). Evidence for extrarenal production of 1 alpha ,25-dihydroxyvitamin D in man. *The Journal of Clinical Investigation, 69*(3), 722-725.

Lapatsanis, D., Moulas, A., Cholevas, V., Soukakos, P., Papadopoulou, Z. L., & Challa, A. (2005). Vitamin D: a necessity for children and adolescents in Greece. *Calcified Tissue International, 77*(6), 348-355.

Lappe, J. M., Travers-Gustafson, D., Davies, K. M., Recker, R. R., & Heaney, R. P. (2007). Vitamin D and calcium supplementation reduces cancer risk: results of a randomized trial. *American Journal of Clinical Nutrition, 85*(6), 1586-1591.

Lark, R., Lester, G., Ontjes, D., Blackwood, A., Hollis, B. W., Hensler, M., et al. (2001). Diminished and eratic absorption of ergocalciferol in adult cystic fibrosis patients. *American Journal of Clinical Nutrition, 73*, 602-606.

Latorre, G. (1961). Effect of overdose of vitamin D_2 on pregnancy in the rat. *Fertility and Sterility, 12*, 343-345.

Lawrence, R. A. (2008). Tackling critical issues for breastfeeding: vitamin D and environmental toxins. *Breastfeeding Medicine, 3*(4), 205.

Leake, C. (1936). Vitamin D toxicity. *California and Western Medicine, 44*(3), 149-150.

Lefkowitz, E., & Garland, C. (1994). Sunlight, vitamin D, and ovarian cancer mortality rates in US women. *International Journal of Epidemiology, 23*, 1133-1136.

Lehtonen-Veromaa, M., Mottonen, T., Irjala, K., Karkkainen, M., Lamberg-Allardt, C., Hakola, P., et al. (1999). Vitamin D intake is low and hypovitaminosis D common in healthy 9-to-15 year old Finnish girls. *European Journal of Clinical Nutrition, 53*, 746-751.

Letterio, J., & Roberts, A. (1997). TGF-b: a critical modulator of immune cell function. *Clin Immunology and Immunopathology, 84*(3), 244-250.

Lieberherr, M. (1987). Effects of vitamin D_3 metabolites on cytosolic free calcium in confluent mouse osteoblasts. *The Journal of Biological Chemistry, 262*(27), 13168-13173.

Lightwood, R. (1932). A case of dwarfism and calcinosis associated with widespread arterial degeneration. *Archives of Diseases in Childhood, 7*, 193.

Lightwood, R., & Payne, W. (1952). Discussion of British Pediatric Association: Proceedings of Twenty-third General Meeting. *Archives of Diseases in Childhood, 27*, 297.

Lin, J., Manson, J. E., Lee, I. M., Cook, N. R., Buring, J. E., & Zhang, S. M. (2007). Intakes of calcium and vitamin D and breast cancer risk in women. *Archives of Internal Medicine, 167*(10), 1050-1059.

Lips, P., Wiersinga, A., Van Ginkel, F. C., Jongen, M. J., Netelenbos, J. C., Hackeng, W. H., et al. (1988). The effect of vitamin D supplementation on vitamin D status and parathyroid function in elderly subjects. *The Journal of Clinical Endocrinology and Metabolism, 67*, 644-650.

Litwiller, R. D., Mattox, V. R., Jardine, I., & et.al. (1982). Evidence for a monoglucuronide of 1,25-dihydroxy-vitamin D_3 in rat bile. *The Journal of Biological Chemistry, 257*, 7491.

Liu, P., Stenger, S., Tang, D., & Modlin, R. (2007). Cutting edge: vitamin D-mediated human antimicrobial activity against Mycobacterium tuberculosis is dependent on the induction of cathelicidin. *Journal of Immunology, 179*, 2060 - 2063.

Liu, P. T., Stenger, S., Li, H., Wenzel, L., Tan, B. H., Krutzik, S. R., et al. (2006). Toll-like receptor triggering of a vitamin D-mediated human antimicrobial response. *Science, 311*(5768), 1770-1773.

Liu, S., Song, Y., Ford, E. S., Manson, J. E., Buring, J. E., & Ridker, P. M. (2005). Dietary calcium, vitamin D, and the prevalence of metabolic syndrome in middle-aged and older U.S. women. *Diabetes Care, 28*(12), 2926-2932.

Lo, C. W., Paris, P. W., & Holick, M. F. (1986). Indian and Pakistani immigrants have the same capacity as Caucasians to produce vitamin D in response to ultraviolet irradiation. *The American Journal of Clinical Nutrition, 44*(5), 683-685.

Looker, A., Dawson-Hughes, B., Calvo, M., Gunter, E., & Sahyoun, N. (2002). Serum 25-hydroxyvitamin D status of adolescents and adults in two seasonal subpopulations from NHANES III. *Bone, 30*(5), 771-777.

Lund, B., & Sorensen, O. H. (1979). Measurement of 25-hydroxyvitamin D in serum and its relation to sunshine, age and vitamin D intake in the Danish population. *Scandinavian Journal of Clinical and Laboratory Investigation, 39*(1), 23-30.

MacLaughlin, J. A., & Holick, M. F. (1983). *Biochemistry and Physiology of the Skin.* New York: Oxford Univ. Press.

MacLaughlin, J. A., & Holick, M. F. (1985). Aging decreases the capacity of the skin to produce vitamin D_3. *The Journal of Clinical Investigation, 76*, 1536-1538.

Madhok, T., & DeLuca, H. (1979). Characteristics of the rat liver microsomal enzyme system converting cholecalciferol into 25-hydroxycholecalciferol. Evidence for the participation of cytochrome p-450. *The Biochemical Journal, 184*(3), 491-499.

Madhok, T. C., Schnoes, H. K., & DeLuca, H. F. (1978). Incorporation of oxygen-18 into the 25-position of cholecalciferol by hepatic cholecalciferol 25-hydroxylase. *The Biochemical Journal, 175*(2), 479-482.

Maghbooli, Z., Hossein-Nezhad, A., Shafaei, A., Karimi, F., Madani, F., & Larijani, B. (2007). Vitamin D status in mothers and their newborns in Iran. *BMC Pregnancy and Childbirth, 7*(1), 1.

Mahomed, K., & Gulmezoglu, AM. Vitamin D supplementation in pregnancy (Cochrane Review). In: Cochrane Database of Systematic Reviews. Chicester, UK: John Wiley & Sons, Ltd., 1999. [Last Reviewed: 2009]

Mallet, E., Gugi, B., Brunelle, P., Henocq, A., Basuyau, J. P., & Lemeur, H. (1986). Vitamin D supplementation in pregnancy: A controlled trial of two methods. *Obstetrics and Gynecology, 68*, 300-304.

Mandel, M., Moorthy, B., & Ghazarian, J. (1990). Reciprocal post-translational regulation of renal 1 alpha- and 24-hydroxylases of 25-hydroxyvitamin D_3 by phosphorylation of ferredoxin. mRNA-directed cell-free synthesis and immunoisolation of ferredoxin. *The Biochemical Journal, 266*(2), 385-392.

Mannion, C., Gray-Donald, K., & Koski, K. (2006). Association of low intake of milk and vitamin D during pregnancy with decreased birth weight. *CMAJ, 174*(9), 1273-1277.

Marie, P. J., Cancela, L., LeBoulch, N., & Miravet, L. (1986). Bone changes due to pregnancy and lactation: Influence of vitamin D status. *The American Journal of Physiology, 251*, E400-E406.

Markestad, T., Aksnes, L., Ulstein, M., & Aarskog, D. (1984). 25-Hydroxyvitamin D and 1,25-dihydroxy vitamin D of D_2 and D_3 origin in maternal and umbilical cord serum after vitamin D_2 supplementation in human pregnancy. *The American Journal of Clinical Nutrition, 40*, 1057-1063.

Martineau, A. R., Wilkinson, R. J., Wilkinson, K. A., Newton, S. M., Kampmann, B., Hall, B. M., et al. (2007). A single dose of vitamin D enhances immunity to mycobacteria. *American Journal of Respiratory and Critical Care Medicine, 176*(2), 208-213).

Martínez, J., Bartoli, F., Recaldini, E., Lavanchy, L., & Bianchetti, M. (2006). A taste comparison of two different liquid colecalciferol (Vitamin D_3) preparations in healthy newborns and infants. *Clinical Drug Investigation, 26*(11), 663-665.

Marx, S., Swart, E., Hamstra, A., & Deluca, H. (1980). Normal intrauterine development of the fetus of a woman receiving extraordinarily high doses of 1,25-dihydroxyvitamin D_3. *The Journal of Clinical Endocrinology and Metabolism, 51*, 1138-1142.

Marya, R. K., Rathee, S., Lata, V., & Mudgil, S. (1981). Effects of vitamin D supplementation in pregnancy. *Gynecologic and Obstetric Investigation, 12*, 155-161.

Mathias, R. S. (2000). Rickets in an infant with Williams Syndrome. *Pediatric Nephrology, 14*, 489-492.

Matsuoka, L. Y., Ide, L., Wortsman, J., MacLaughlin, J. A., & Holick, M. F. (1987). Sunscreens suppress cutaneous vitamin D_3 synthesis. *The Journal of Clinical Endocrinology and Metabolism, 64*(6), 1165-1168.

Matsuoka, L. Y., Wortsman, J., Dannenberg, M. J., Hollis, B. W., Lu, Z., & Holick, M. F. (1992). Clothing prevents ultraviolet-B-radiation-dependent photosynthesis of vitamin D_3. *The Journal of Clinical Endocrinology and Metabolism, 75*, 1099-1103.

Matsuoka, L. Y., Wortsman, J., Haddad, J. G., & Hollis, B. W. (1989). *In vivo* threshold for cutaneous synthesis of vitamin D_3. *The Journal of Laboratory and Clinical Medicine, 114*, 301-305.

Matsuoka, L. Y., Wortsman, J., Haddad, J. G., & Hollis, B. W. (1990). Skin types and epidermal photosynthesis of vitamin D_3. *Journal of the American Academy of Dermatology, 23*(3), 525-526.

Matsuoka, L. Y., Wortsman, J., Haddad, J. G., Kolm, P., & Hollis, B. W. (1991). Racial pigmentation and the cutaneous synthesis of vitamin D. *Archives of Dermatology, 127*, 536-538.

Matsuoka, L. Y., Wortsman, J., Hanifan, N., & Holick, M. F. (1988). Chronic sunscreen use decreases circulating concentrations of 25-hydroxyvitamin D: A preliminary study. *Archives of Dermatology, 124*, 1802-1804.

Matsuoka, L. Y., Wortsman, J., & Hollis, B. W. (1988). Lack of effect of exogenous calcitriol on cutaneous production of vitamin D_3. *The Journal of Clinical Endocrinology and Metabolism, 66*, 451-453.

Matsuoka, L. Y., Wortsman, J., & Hollis, B. W. (1990a). Suntanning and cutaneous synthesis of vitamin D_3. *The Journal of Laboratory and Clinical Medicine, 116*, 87-90.

Matsuoka, L. Y., Wortsman, J., & Hollis, B. W. (1990b). Use of topical sunscreen for the evaluation of regional synthesis of vitamin D_3. *Journal of the American Academy of Dermatology, 22*, 772-775.

Mawer, E. B., Backhouse, J., Holman, C. A., Lumb, G. A., & Stanbury, S. W. (1972). The distribution and storage of vitamin D and its metabolites in human tissues. *Clinical Science, 43*(3), 413-431.

Mawer, E. B., Schaefer, K., Lumb, G. A., & Stanbury, S. W. (1971). The metabolism of isotopically labelled vitamin D_3 in man: the influence of the state of vitamin D nutrition. *Clinical Science, 40*(1), 39-53.

Maxwell, J. D., Ang, L., Brooke, O. G., & Brown, I. R. F. (1981). Vitamin D supplements enhance weight gain and nutrional status in pregnant Asians. *British Journal of Obstetrics and Gynaecology, 88*, 987-991.

Mayer, J. (1957). Armand Trousseau and the arrow of time. *Nutrition Reviews, 15*, 321-323.

McCollum, E. (1957). *A history of nutrition.* Cambridge, MA: Riverside Press.

McCollum, E. (1964). *From Kansas farm boy to scientist.* Lawrence, KS: University of Kansas Press.

McCollum, E. V., Simmonds, N., Becket, J. E., & Shipley, P. G. (1922). Studies on experimental rickets. XXI. An experimental demonstration of the existence of a vitamin, which promotes calcium deposition. *The Journal of Biological Chemistry, 53*(8), 219-312.

McDonnell, D. P., Mangelsdorf, D. J., Pike, J. W., Haussler, M. R., & O'Malley, B. W. (1987). Molecular cloning of complementary DNA encoding the avian receptor for vitamin D. *Science, 235*(4793), 1214-1217.

McGill, A. T., Stewart, J. M., Lithander, F. E., Strik, C. M., & Poppitt, S. D. (2008). Relationships of low serum vitamin D_3 with anthropometry and markers of the metabolic syndrome and diabetes in overweight and obesity. *Nutrition Journal, 7*, 4.

McGrath, J. (1999). Hypothesis: is low prenatal vitamin D a risk-modifying factor for schizophrenia? *Schizophrenia Research, 49*, 173-177.

McGrath, J. (2001). Does "imprinting" with low prenatal vitamin D contribute to the risk of various adult disorders? *Medical Hypothesis, 56*, 367-371.

McGrath, J., Feton, F., & Eyles, D. (2001). Does "imprinting" with low prenatal vitamin D contribute to the risk of various adult disorders? *Medical Hypothesis, 56*, 367-371.

McGrath, J., Selten, J. P., & Chant, D. (2002). Long-term trends in sunshine duration and its association with schizophrenia birth rates and age at first registration-data from Australia and the Netherlands. *Schizophrenia Research, 54*, 199-212.

Mead Johnson Nutrition. (2004). *Mead Johnson nutritional product handbook.* Evansville: Mead Johnson and Company.

Meier, C., Woitge, H., Witte, K., Lemmer, B., & Seibel, M. (2004). Supplementation with oral vitamin D_3 and calcium during winter prevents seasonal bone loss: A randomized controlled open-label prospective trial. *Journal of Bone and Mineral Researcj, 19*, 1221-1230.

Mellanby, E. (1919). An experimental investigation of rickets. *Lancet, 1*, 407-412.

Mellanby, E. (1921). Experimental rickets. *Medical Research (Great Britain). Special Report Series, SRS-61*, 1-78.

Mellanby, E., & Cantag, M. (1919). Experimental investigation of rickets. *Lancet, 196*, 407-412.

Merke, J., Klaus, G., Hugel, U., Waldherr, R., & Ritz, E. (1986). No 1,25-dihydroxyvitamin D_3 receptors on osteoclasts of calcium-deficient chicken despite demonstrable receptors on circulating monocytes. *The Journal of Clinical Investigation, 77*(1), 312-314.

Merlino, L. A., Curtis, J., Mikuls, T. R., Cerhan, J. R., Criswell, L. A., & Saag, K. G. (2004). Vitamin D intake is inversely associated with rheumatoid arthritis: results from the Iowa Women's Health Study. *Arthritis and Rheumatism, 50*(1), 72-77.

Mikhak, B., Hunter, D. J., Spiegelman, D., Platz, E. A., Hollis, B. W., & Giovannucci, E. (2007). Vitamin D receptor (VDR) gene polymorphisms and haplotypes, interactions with plasma 25-hydroxyvitamin D and 1,25-dihydroxyvitamin D, and prostate cancer risk. *Prostate, 67*(9), 911-923.

Misra, M., Pacaud, D., Petryk, A., Collett-Solberg, P. F., & Kappy, M. (2008). Vitamin D deficiency in children and its management: review of current knowledge and recommendations. *Pediatrics, 122*(2), 398-417.

Molgaard, C., & Michaelsen, K. (2003). Vitamin D and bone health in early life. *Proceedings of the National Academy of Sciences in the United States of America, 62*(4), 823-828.

Moncrieff, M., & Fadahunsi, T. O. (1974). Congenital rickets due to maternal vitamin D deficiency. *Archives of Diseases in Childhood, 49*(10), 810-811.

Monks, J., Huey, P., Hanson, L., Eckel, R., Neville, M., & Gavigan, S. (2001). A lipoprotein-containing particle is transferred from the serum across the mammary epithelium into the milk of lactating mice. *Journal of Lipid Research, 42*, 686-696.

Mordan-McCombs, S., Valrance, M., Zinser, G., Tenniswood, M., & Welsh, J. (2007). Calcium, vitamin D and the vitamin D receptor: impact on prostate and breast cancer in preclinical models. *Nutrition Reviews, 65*(8 Pt 2), S131-133.

Morgan, V., McGrath, J., Hultman, C., Zubrick, S., Bower, C., Valuri, G., et al. (2009). The offspring of women with severe mental disorder. In J. P. Newnham & M. G. Ross (Eds.), *Early Life Origins of Human Health and Disease* (pp. 202-204). Basel: S. Karger AG.

Morris, C. A., & Mervis, C. B. (2000). William's syndrome and related disorders. *Annual Review of Genomics and Human Genetics, 1*, 461-484.

Morris, G. S., Zhou, Q., Hegsted, M., & Keenan, M. J. (1995). Maternal consumption of a low vitamin D diet retards metabolic and contractile development in the neonatal rat heart. *Journal of Molecular and Cellular Cardiology, 27*(1745-50).

Mozolowski, W. (1939). Jedrzej Sniadecki (1768-1883) on the cure of rickets. *Nature, 143*, 121.

Munger, K., Zhang, S., O'Reilly, E., Hernan, M., Olek, M., Willett, W., et al. (2004). Vitamin D intake and incidence of multiple sclerosis. *Neurology, 62*, 60-65.

Munger, K. L., Levin, L. I., Hollis, B. W., Howard, N. S., & Ascherio, A. (2006). Serum 25-hydroxyvitamin D levels and risk of multiple sclerosis. *JAMA, 296*(23), 2832-2838.

Mylott, B., Kump, T, Bolton, ML, Greenbaum, LA. (2004). Rickets in the Dairy State. *WMJ, 103*(5), 84-87.

Nagubandi, S., Kumar, R., Londowski, J. M., Corradino, R. A., & Tietz, P. S. (1980). Role of vitamin D glucosiduronate in calcium homeostasis. *The Journal of Clinical Investigation, 66*(6), 1274-1280.

Najada, A., Habashneh, M., & Khader, M. (2004). The frequency of nutritional rickets among hospitalized infants and its relation to respiratory diseases. *Journal of Tropical Pediatrics, 50*(6), 364-368.

Nakamura, T., Suzuki, K., Hirai, T., Kurokawa, T., & Orimo, H. (1992). Increased bone volume and reduced bone turnover in vitamin D-replete rabbits by the administration of 24R,25-dihydroxyvitamin D$_3$. *Bone, 13*(3), 229-236.

Narang, N., Gupta, R., Jain, M., & Aaronson, K. (1984). Role of vitamin D in pulmonary tuberculosis. *The Journal of the Association of Physicians of India, 32*, 185-186.

National Academy of Sciences. (1989). *Recommended dietary allowances.* (10th edition ed.). Washington, D.C.: National Academy Press.

National Coalition for Skin Cancer Prevention. (1998). *The national forum for skin cancer prevention in health, physical education, recreation and youth sports.* Reston, VA: American Association for Health Education.

Nebel, L., & Ornoy, A. (1966). Effect of hypervitaminosis D_2 on fertility and pregnancy in rats. *Israel Journal of Medical Sciences, 2,* 14-21.

Nebel, L., & Ornoy, A. (1971). Structural alterations in rat placenta following hypervitaminosis D_2. *Israel Journal of Medical Sciences, 7,* 647-655.

Neiderhoffer, N., Bobryshev, Y. V., Laftaud-Idjouadiene, I., Giummelly, P., & Atkinson, J. (1997). Aortic calcification produced by vitamin D_3 plus nicotine. *Journal of Vascular Research, 34,* 386-398.

Nemani, R., Ghazarian, J., Moorthy, B., Wongsurawat, N., Strong, R., & Armbrecht, H. (1989). Phosphorylation of ferredoxin and regulation of renal mitochondrial 25-hydroxyvitamin D-1 alpha-hydroxylase activity *in vitro. The Journal of Biological Chemistry, 264*(26), 15361-15366.

Nesby-O'Dell, S., Scanlon, K., Cogswell, M., Gillespie, C., Hollis, B., Looker, A., et al. (2002). Hypovitaminosis D prevalence and determinants among African American and white women of reproductive age: Third National Health and Nutrition Examination Survey: 1988-1994. *The American Journal of Clinical Nutrition, 76,* 187-192.

NIH. (2003). *Vitamin D and Health in the 21st Century: Bone and Beyond.* Bethesda, Maryland.

Norman, P., Moss, I., Sian, M., Gosling, M., & Powell, J. (2002). Maternal and postnatal vitamin D ingestion influences rat aortic structure function and elastin content. *Cardiovascular Research, 55,* 369-374.

Nozza, J. M., & Rodda, C. P. (2001). Vitamin D deficiency in mothers of infants with rickets. *The Medical Journal of Australia, 175*(5), 253-255.

O'Loan, J., Eyles, D. W., Kesby, J., Ko, P., McGrath, J. J., & Burne, T. H. J. (2007). Vitamin D deficiency during various stages of pregnancy in the rat; its impact on development and behaviour in adult offspring. *Psychoneuroendocrinology, 32*(3), 227-234.

O'Riordan, J. L. (2006). Rickets in the 17th century. *Journal of Bone and Mineral Research, 21*(10), 1506-1510.

Ohyama, Y., Noshiro, M., & Okuda, K. (1991). Cloning and expression of cDNA encoding 25-hydroxyvitamin D_3 24-hydroxylase. *FEBS Letters, 278*(2), 195-198.

Oliveri, M. B., Ladizesky, M., Mautalen, C. A., Alonso, A., & Martinez, L. (1993). Seasonal variations of 25 hydroxyvitamin D and parathyroid hormone in Ushuaia (Argentina), the southernmost city of the world. *Bone and Mineral, 20*(1), 99-108.

Olmez, D., Bober, E., Buyukgebiz, A., & Cimrin, D. (2006). The frequency of vitamin D insufficiency in healthy female adolescents. *Acta Paediatrica, 95,* 1266-1269.

Olson, E. B., Jr., Knutson, J. C., Bhattacharyya, M. H., & DeLuca, H. F. (1976). The effect of hepatectomy on the synthesis of 25-hydroxyvitamin D_3. *The Journal of Clinical Investigation, 57*(5), 1213-1220.

Omdahl, J., Holick, M., Suda, T., Tanaka, Y., & DeLuca, H. F. (1971). Biological activity of 1,25-dihydroxycholecalciferol. *Biochemistry, 10*(15), 2935-2940.

Onisko, B., Esvelt, R., Schnoes, H., & DeLuca, H. (1980). Metabolites of 1 alpha, 25-dihydroxyvitamin D_3 in rat. *Biochemistry, 19*(17), 4124-4130.

Ornoy, A., & Nebel, L. (1967). Alterations in the mineral composition and metabolism of rat fetuses and their placenta induced by maternal hypervitaminosis D₂. *Israel Journal of Medical Sciences, 4*, 827-833.

Ornoy, A., & Nebel, L. (1970). Effects of hypervitaminosis D₂ altered by pregnancy in rats. *Israel Journal of Medical Sciences, 6*(622-629).

Ornoy, A., Nebel, L., & Menczel, J. (1969). Impaired osteogenesis and ossification of fetal long bones induced by maternal hypervitaminosis D in rats. *Archives of Pathology, 87*, 563-570.

Otani, T., Iwasaki, M., Sasazuki, S., Inoue, M., & Tsugane, S. (2007). Plasma vitamin D and risk of colorectal cancer: the Japan Public Health Center-Based Prospective Study. *British Journal of Cancer, 97*(3), 446-451.

Palm, T. (1890). The geographical distribution and aetiology of rickets. *Practitioner, 45*, 270-279, 321-342.

Park, E. (1923). The etiology of rickets. *Physiological Reviews, 3*, 106-119.

Park, E. A. (1940). The therapy of rickets. *JAMA, 115*(5), 370-379.

Pawley, N., & Bishop, N. (2004). Prenatal and infant predictors of bone health: the influence of vitamin D. *The American Journal of Clinical Nutrition, 80*(suppl), 1748S-1751S.

Pettifor, J. (2005). Rickets and vitamin D deficiency in children and adolescents. *Endocrinology and Metabolism Clinics of North America, 34*(3), 537-553.

Pfannenstiel. (1927). *Klin Woch, 6*, 2310.

Pittard, W. B., Geddes, K. M., Hulsey, T. C., & Hollis, B. W. (1991). How much vitamin D for neonates? *American Journal of Diseases of Children, 145*, 1147-1149.

Pittas, A. G., Dawson-Hughes, B., Li, T., Van Dam, R. M., Willett, W. C., Manson, J. E., et al. (2006). Vitamin D and calcium intake in relation to type 2 diabetes in women. *Diabetes Care, 29*(3), 650-656.

Pittas, A. G., Harris, S. S., Stark, P. C., & Dawson-Hughes, B. (2007). The effects of calcium and vitamin D supplementation on blood glucose and markers of inflammation in nondiabetic adults. *Diabetes Care, 30*(4), 980-986.

Pittas, A. G., Lau, J., Hu, F. B., & Dawson-Hughes, B. (2007). The role of vitamin D and calcium in type 2 diabetes. A systematic review and meta-analysis. *Journal of Clinical Endocrinology and Metabolism, 92*(6).

Platz, E. A., Leitzmann, M. F., Hollis, B. W., Willett, W. C., & Giovannucci, E. (2004). Plasma 1,25-dihydroxy- and 25-hydroxyvitamin D and subsequent risk of prostate cancer. *Cancer Causes and Control, 15*, 255-265.

Plotnikoff, G., & Quigley, J. (2003). Prevalence of severe hypovitaminosis D in patients with persistent, nonspecific musculoskeletal pain. *Mayo Clinic Proceedings, 78*, 1463-1470.

Polskin, L. J., Kramer, B., & Sobel, A. E. (1945). Selection of vitamin D in milks of women fed fish liver oil. *The Journal of Nutrition, 30*, 451-466.

Ponsonby, A., Lucas, R., & vanderMei, I. (2005). UVR, vitamin D and three autoimmune diseases--multiple sclerosis, type 1 diabetes, rheumatoid arthritis. *Photochemistry and Photobiology, 81*, 1267 - 1275.

Portale, A. A., Booth, B. E., Halloran, B. P., & Morris, R. C., Jr. (1984). Effect of dietary phosphorus on circulating concentrations of 1,25-dihydroxyvitamin D and immunoreactive parathyroid hormone in children with moderate renal insufficiency. *The Journal of Clinical Investigation, 73*(6), 1580-1589.

Poulter, L. W., Rook, G. A., Steele, J., & Condez, A. (1987). Influence of 1,25-(OH)2 vitamin D_3 and gamma interferon on the phenotype of human peripheral blood monocyte-derived macrophages. *Infection and Immununity, 55*(9), 2017-2020.

Prentice, A., Jarjou, L. M., Goldberg, G. R., Bennett, J., Cole, T. J., & Schoenmakers, I. (2009). Maternal plasma 25-hydroxyvitamin D concentration and birthweight, growth and bone mineral accretion of Gambian infants. *Acta Paediatrica, 98*(8), 1360-1362.

Pugliese, M. T., Blumberg, D. L., Hludzinski, J., & Kay, S. (1998). Nutritional rickets in suburbia. *Journal of the American College of Nutrition, 17*(6), 637-641.

Rajakumar, K. (2003). Vitamin D, cod-liver oil, sunlight, and rickets: A historical perspective. *Pediatrics, 112*(2), e132-135.

Rajakumar, K., & Thomas, S. B. (2005). Reemerging nutritional rickets: A historical perspective. *Archives of Pediatrics & Adolescent Medicine, 159*(4), 335-341.

Rao, R. K. (1990). Prospective study of colorectal cancer in the West of Scotland: 10-year follow-up. *The British Journal of Surgery, 77*(12), 1434.

Rao, R. K. (2002). Prostate cancer. *Tropical Doctor, 32*(3), 155-157.

Reeve, L. E., Chesney, R. W., & Deluca, H. F. (1982). Vitamin D of human milk: Identification of biologically active forms. *The American Journal of Clinical Nutrition, 26*, 122-126.

Rehman, P. (1994). Sub-clinical rickets and recurrent infection. *Journal of Tropical Pediatrics, 40*, 58.

Reichel, H., Koeffler, H. P., & Norman, A. W. (1989). The role of the vitamin D endocrine system in health and disease. *The New England Journal of Medicine, 320*(15), 980-991.

Reichel, H., & Norman, A. W. (1989). Systemic effects of vitamin D. *Annual Review of Medicine, 40*, 71-78.

Robien, K., Cutler, G. J., & Lazovich, D. (2007). Vitamin D intake and breast cancer risk in postmenopausal women: the Iowa Women's Health Study. *Cancer Causes & Control, 18*(7), 775-782.

Robinson, B. G., Clifton-Bligh, P., Posen, S., & Morris, B. J. (1983). Plasma vasopressin in hypercalcaemic states. *Australian and New Zealand Journal of Medicine, 13*(1), 5-7.

Rohan, T. (2007). Epidemiological studies of vitamin D and breast cancer. *Nutrition Reviews, 65*(8 Pt 2), S80-83.

Rook, G. (1986). Vitamin D and tuberculosis. *Tubercle, 67*(2), 155-156.

Rook, G. A. (1988). The role of vitamin D in tuberculosis. *The American Review of Respiratory Disease, 138*(4), 768-770.

Rook, G. A., & Steele, J. (1987). Macrophage regulation of vitamin D_3 metabolites. *Nature, 326*(6108), 21-22.

Rook, G. A., Steele, J., Fraher, L., Barker, S., Karmali, R., O'Riordan, J., et al. (1986). Vitamin D_3, gamma interferon, and control of proliferation of Mycobacterium tuberculosis by human monocytes. *Immunology, 57*(1), 159-163.

Rook, G. A., Taverne, J., Leveton, C., & Steele, J. (1987). The role of gamma-interferon, vitamin D$_3$ metabolites and tumour necrosis factor in the pathogenesis of tuberculosis. *Immunology, 62*(2), 229-234.

Rosen, H., Reshef, A., Maeda, N., Lippoldt, A., Shpizen, S., Triger, L., et al. (1998). Markedly reduced bile acid synthesis but maintained levels of cholesterol and vitamin D metabolites in mice with disrupted sterol 27-hydroxylase gene. *The Journal of Biological Chemistry, 273*(24), 14805-14812.

Rosen, J. F., Roginsky, M., Nathenson, G., & Finberg, L. (1974). 25-Hydroxyvitamin D. Plasma levels in mothers and their premature infants with neonatal hypocalcemia. *American Journal of Diseases of Children, 127*(2), 220-223.

Roth, D. E., Jones, A. B., Prosser, C., Robinson, J. L., & Vohra, S. (2009). Vitamin D status is not associated with the risk of hospitalization for acute bronchiolitis in early childhood. *European Journal of Clinical Nutrition, 63,* 2, 297-299.

Rothberg, A. D., Pettifor, J. M., Cohen, D. F., Sonnendecker, E. W., & Ross, F. P. (1982). Maternal-infant vitamin D relationships during breast-feeding. *The Journal of Pediatrics, 101*(4), 500-503.

Ruhrah, J. (1925). *Pedatrics of the past.* New York, NY: Paul B. Hoeber, Inc.

Russell, A., & Young, W. (1954). Severe infantile hypercalcaemia. Long-term response of 2 cases to low calcium diet. *Proceedings of the Royal Society of Medicine, 47*(1035), 37-42.

Saadi, H. F., Dawodu, A., Afandi, B. O., Zayed, R., Benedict, S., & Nagelkerke, N. (2007). Efficacy of daily and monthly high-dose calciferol in vitamin D-deficient nulliparous and lactating women. *The American Journal of Clinical Nutrition, 85*(6), 1565-1571.

Safadi, F. F., Thornton, P., Magiera, H., & et.al. (1999). Osteopathy and resistance to vitamin D toxicity in mice null for vitamin D binding protein. *The Journal of Clinical Investigation, 103*, 239.

Sahshi, Y., Suzuki, T., Higaki, M., & Asano, T. (1967). Metabolism of vitamin D in animals: Isolation of vitamin D-sulfate from mammalian milk. *The Journal of Vitaminology, 13*, 33-36.

Scanlon, K. S. (2001). *Vitamin D Expert Panel Meeting, October 11-12, 2001.* Paper presented at the Center for Disease Control, Atlanta, GA. Retrieved February 11, 2010 from *http://www.cdc.gov/nccdphp/dnpa/nutrition/pdf/Vitamin_D_Expert_Panel_Meeting.pdf.*

Schleithoff, S. S., Zittermann, A., Stuttgen, B., Tenderich, G., Berthold, H. K., Korfer, R., et al. (2003). Low serum levels of intact osteocalcin in patients with congestive heart failure. *Journal of Bone and Mineral Metabolism, 21*(4), 247-252.

Schleithoff, S. S., Zittermann, A., Tenderich, G., Berthold, H. K., Stehle, P., & Koerfer, R. (2006). Vitamin D supplementation improves cytokine profiles in patients with congestive heart failure: a double-blind, randomized, placebo-controlled trial. *The American Journal of Clinical Nutrition, 83*(4), 754-759.

Schlesinger, B., Butler, N., & Black, J. (1956). Severe type of infantile hypercalcaemia. *The British Journal of Nutrition, 1*(4959), 127-134.

Schnadower, D., Agarwal, C., Oberfield, S., Fennoy, I., & Pusic, M. (2006). Hypocalcemic seizures and secondary bilateral femoral fractures in an adolescent with primary vitamin D deficiency. *Pediatrics, 118*(5), 22226-22230.

Schwartz, Z., Bonewald, L. F., Caulfield, K., Brooks, B., & Boyan, B. D. (1993). Direct effects of transforming growth factor-beta on chondrocytes are modulated by vitamin D metabolites in a cell maturation-specific manner. *Endocrinology, 132*(4), 1544-1552.

Seelig, M. (1969). Vitamin D and cardiovascular, renal and brain damage in infancy and childhood. *Annals of the New York Academy of Sciences, 147*, 537-582.

Senator, H. (1877). *Cyclopedia of the practice of medicine* (Vol. XVI). New York: William Wood.

Shehadeh, N., Shamir, R., Berant, M., & Etzioni, A. (2001). Insulin in human milk and the prevention of type 1 diabetes. *Pediatric Diabetes, 2*(4), 175-177.

Sher, E., Eisman, J. A., Moseley, J. M., & Martin, T. J. (1981). Whole-cell uptake and nuclear localization of 1,25-dihydroxycholecalciferol by breast cancer cells (T47 D) in culture. *The Biochemical Journal, 200*(2), 315-320.

Sherman, S. S., Hollis, B. W., & Tobin, J. D. (1990). Vitamin D status and related parameters in a healthy population: the effects of age, sex, and season. *The Journal of Clinical Endocrinology and Metabolism, 71*(2), 405-413.

Shipley, P., Park, E., McCollum, E., Simmonds, N., & Parsons, H. (1921). Studies on experimental rickets. II. The effect of cod liver oil administered to rats with experimental rickets. *The Journal of Biological Chemistry, XLV*, 343-350.

Sills, I., Skuza, KA, Horlick, MN, Schwartz, MS, Rapaport, R. (1994). Vitamin D deficiency rickets: reports of its demise are exaggerated. *Clinical Pediatrics (Phila), 33*(8), 491-493.

Smith, J. E., & Goodman, D. S. (1971). The turnover and transport of vitamin D and of a polar metabolite with the properties of 25-hydroxycholecalciferol in human plasma. *The Journal of Clinical Investigation, 50*(10), 2159-2167.

Smith, R., & Dent, C. E. (1969). Vitamin D requirements in adults. Clinical and metabolic studies on seven patients with nutritional osteomalacia. *Bibliotheca Nutritio et Dieta, 13*, 44-45.

Soliman, A. T., El-Dabbagh, M., Adel, A., Ali, M. A., Aziz Bedair, E. M., & Elalaily, R. K. (2010). Clinical responses to a mega-dose of vitamin D_3 in infants and toddlers with vitamin d deficiency rickets. *Journal of Tropical Pediatrics, 56*(1), 19-26.

Specker, B. L., Ho, M. L., Oestreich, A., Yin, T. A., Shui, Q. M., Chen, X. C., et al. (1992). Prospective study of vitamin D supplementation and rickets in China. *The Journal of Pediatrics, 120*(5), 733-739.

Specker, B. L., Tsang, R. C., & Hollis, B. W. (1985). Effect of race and diet on human milk vitamin D and 25(OH)D. *American Journal of Diseases of Children, 139*, 1134-1137.

Specker, B. L., Valanis, B., Hertzberg, V., Edwards, N., & Tsang, R. C. (1985). Sunshine exposure and serum 25-hydroxyvitamin D concentrations in exclusively breast-fed infants. *The Journal of Pediatrics, 107*(3), 372-376.

St-Arnaud, R., Arabian, A., Travers, R., Barletta, F., Raval-Pandya, M., Chapin, K., et al. (2000). Deficient Mineralization of Intramembranous Bone in Vitamin D-24-Hydroxylase-Ablated Mice Is Due to Elevated 1,25-Dihydroxyvitamin D and Not to the Absence of 24,25-Dihydroxyvitamin D. *Endocrinology, 141*(7), 2658-2666.

Stamp, T. C., Haddad, J. G., & Twigg, C. A. (1977). Comparison of oral 25(OH)D_3, vitamin D, and ultraviolet light as determinants of circulating 25(OH)D. *Lancet, 1*, 1341-1343.

Standing Committee on the Scientific Evaluation of Dietary Reference Intakes Food and Nutrition Board, I. o. M. (1997). *Calcium, phosphorus, magnesium, vitamin D and fluoride.* Washington, DC: National Academy Press.

Stearns, G., & Jeans, P. (1936). The effect of vitamin D on linear growth in infancy. *The Journal of Pediatrics, 9*, 1-10.

Steenbock, H. (1924). The induction of growth promoting and calcifying properties in a ration by exposure to light. *Science, 60,* 224-225.

Steenbock, H., & Black, A. (1924). Fat-soluble vitamins. XVII. The induction of gorwth-promoting and calcifying propeties in a ration by exposure to ultra-violet light. *The Journal of Biological Chemistry, 61,* 405-422.

Steenbock, H., & Nelson, M. (1924). Fat-soluble vitamins. XIX. The induction of calcifying properties in a rickets-producing ration by radiant energy. *Methods in Enzymology, 62,* 209-216.

Still, G. (1931). *The History of pediatrics. The progress of the study of children up to the end of the XVIIIth century.* London, United Kingdom: Oxford University Press, Humphrey Milford.

Stumpf, W. E., Clark, S. A., O'Brien , L. P., & Reid, F. A. (1988). $1,25(OH)_2D_3$ sites of action in spinal cord and sensory ganglion. *Anatomy and Embryology, 177,* 307-310.

Stumpf, W. E., Clark, S. A., Sar, M., & DeLuca, H. F. (1984). Topographical and developmental studies on target sites of 1,25 (OH)2 vitamin D_3 in skin. *Cell and Tissue Research, 238*(3), 489-496.

Stumpf, W. E., Sar, M., Reid, F. A., Tanaka, Y., & DeLuca, H. F. (1979). Target cells for 1,25-dihydroxyvitamin D_3 in intestinal tract, stomach, kidney, skin, pituitary, and parathyroid. *Science, 206*(4423), 1188-1190.

Taha, S. A., Dost, S. M., & Sedrani, S. H. (1984). 25(OH)D and total calcium: Extraordinarily low plasma concentrations in Saudi mothers and their neonates. *Pediatric Research, 18,* 739-741.

Takeuchi, A., Okano, T., Tsugawa, H., Tasaka, Y., Koboyashi, T., Kodama, S., et al. (1989). Effects of ergocalciferol supplementation on the concentration of vitamin D and its metabolites in human milk. *The Journal of Nutrition, 119,* 1639-1646.

Takigawa, M., Enomoto, M., Shirai, E., Nishii, Y., & Suzuki, F. (1988). Differential effects of l{alpha},25-dihydroxycholecalciferol and 24r,25-dihydroxycholecalciferol on the proliferation and the differentiated phenotype of rabbit costal chondrocytes in culture. *Endocrinology, 122*(3), 831-839.

Tanaka, Y., DeLuca, H. F., Omdahl, J., & Holick, M. F. (1971). Mechanism of action of 1,25-dihydroxycholecalciferol on intestinal calcium transport. *Proceedings of the National Academy of Sciences in the United States of America, 68*(6), 1286-1288.

Tanaka, Y., Frank, H., & Deluca, H. F. (1973). Biological activity of $1,25(OH)_2D_3$ in the rat. *Endocrinology, 92,* 417-422.

Tanner, J. T., Smith, J., Defibaugh, P., Angyal, G., Villalobos, M., Bueno, M. P., et al. (1988). Survey of vitamin content of fortified milk. *Journal - Association of Official Analytical Chemists, 71*(3), 607-610.

Taussig, H. B. (1966). Possible injury to the cardiovascular system from vitamin D. *Annals of Internal Medicine, 65,* 1195-1200.

Taylor, S. N., Wagner, C. L., & Hollis, B. W. (2008). Vitamin D supplementation during lactation to support infant and mother. *Journal of the American College of Nutrition, 27*(6), 690-701.

The EURODIAB Substudy 2 Study Group. (1999). Vitamin D supplement in early childhood and risk for Type 1 (insulin-dependent) diabetes mellitus. *Diabetologia, 42,* 51-54.

Thomas, M. K., Lloyd-Jones, D. M., Thadhani, R. I., Shaw, A. C., Deraska, D. J., Kitch, B. T., et al. (1998). Hypovitaminosis D in medical inpatients. *The New England Journal of Medicine, 338,* 777-783.

Toda, T., Toda, Y., & Kummerow, F. A. (1985). Coronary arterial lesions in piglets from sows fed moderate excessess of vitamin of vitamin D. *The Tohoku Journal of Experimental Medicine, 145,* 303-310.

Tomashek, K. M., Nesby, S., Scanlon, K. S., Cogswell, M. E., Powell, K. E., Parashar, U. D., et al. (2001). Nutritional rickets in Georgia. *Pediatrics, 107*(4), E45.

Trousseau, A. (1872). *Lectures on clinical medicine, delivered at the Hotel Dieu. Translated by Sir John Cormack* (S. J. Cormack, Trans. 3rd ed.). London: New Sydenham Society.

*Tseng, M., Breslow, R. A., Graubard, B. I., & Ziegler, R. G. (2005). Dairy, calcium, and vitamin D intakes and prostate cancer risk in the National Health and Nutrition Examination Epidemiologic Follow-up Study cohort. *The American Journal of Clinical Nutrition, 81*(5), 1147-1154.

Tucker, G., 3rd, Gagnon, R. E., & Haussler, M. R. (1973). Vitamin D 3 -25-hydroxylase: tissue occurrence and apparent lack of regulation. *Archives of Biochemistry and Biophysics, 155*(1), 47-57.

Turner, R. T., Avioli, R. C., & Bell, N. H. (1984). Extrarenal metabolism of 25-hydroxycholecalciferol in the rat: regulation by 1,25-dihydroxycholecalciferol. *Calcified Tissue International, 36*(3), 274-278.

van der Meer, I., Karamali, N., & Boeke, A. (2006). High prevalence of vitamin D deficiency in pregnant non-Western women the The Hague, Netherlands. *The American Journal of Clinical Nutrition, 84,* 350-353.

Veenstra, T. D., Prufer, K., Keonigsberger, C., Brimijoin , S. W., Grande, J. P., & Kumar, R. (1998). 1,25-dihydroxyvitamin D_3 receptors in the central nervous system of the rat embryo. *Brain Research, 4,* 193-205.

Vicchio, D., Yergey, A., O'Brien, K., Allen, L., Ray, R., & Holick, M. (1993). Quantification and kinetics of 25-hydroxyvitamin D_3 by isotope dilution liquid chromatography/thermospray mass spectrometry. *Biological Mass Spectrometry, 22*(1), 53-58.

Vieth, R. (1990). The mechanisms of vitamin D toxicity. *Bone and Mineral, 11*(3), 267-272.

Vieth, R. (1999). Vitamin D supplementation, 25-hydroxy-vitamin D concentrations, and safety. *The American Journal of Clinical Nutrition, 69,* 842-856.

Vieth, R. (2009a). How to optimize vitamin D supplementation to prevent cancer, based on cellular adaptation and hydroxylase enzymology. *Anticancer Research, 29*(9), 3675-3684.

Vieth, R. (2009b). Vitamin D and cancer mini-symposium: the risk of additional vitamin D. *Annals of Epidemiology, 19*(7), 441-445.

Vieth, R., Bischoff-Ferrari, H., Boucher, B., Dawson-Hughes, B., Garland, C., Heaney, R., et al. (2007). The urgent need to recommend an intake of vitamin D that is effective. *The American Journal of Clinical Nutrition, 85,* 649 - 650.

Vieth, R., Chan, P. C. R., & MacFarlane, G. D. (2001). Efficacy and safety of vitamin D_3 intake exceeding the lowest observed adverse effect level (LOAEL). *The American Journal of Clinical Nutrition, 73*(2), 288-294.

Vieth, R., Cole, D., Hawker, G., Trang, H., & Rubin, L. (2001). Wintertime vitamin D insufficiency is common in young Canadian women, and their vitamin D intake does not prevent it. *European Journal of Clinical Nutrition, 55,* 1091-1097.

Vieth, R., Ladak, Y., & Walfish, P. (2003). Age-related changes in the 25-hydroxyvitamin D versus parathyroid hormone relationship suggest a different reason why older adults require more vitamin D. *The Journal of Clinical Endocrinology and Metabolism, 88,* 185-191.

Vieth, R., Pinto, T. R., Reen, B. S., & Wong, M. M. (2002). Vitamin D poisoning by table sugar. *Lancet, 359*(9307), 672.

Vitamin D supplementation: Recommendations for Canadian mothers and infants. (2007). *Paediatrics & Child Health, 12*(7), 583-598.

Wagner, C., Johnson, D., Hulsey, T., Ebeling, M., Shary, J., Smith, P., et al. (2010b). Vitamin D supplementation during pregnancy part 2 NICHD/CTSA Randomized Clinical Trial (RCT): Outcomes. *Pediatric Research, in press*([abstract]).

Wagner, C., Johnson, D., Hulsey, T., Hamilton, S., McNeil, B., Davis, D., et al. (2008). Vitamin D deficiency (VDD) during pregnancy: At epidemic proportions in SC (abstract). *Pediatric Research*.

Wagner, C. l., McNeil, R., Hamilton, S., Davis, D., Prudgen, C., Winkler, J., et al. (2010). Vitamin D (vitD) supplementation during pregnancy: Thrasher Research Fund RCT in SC community health center networks. *Pediatric Research, in press*([abstract]).

Wagner, C. L., Greer, F. R., & American Academy of Pediatrics, Section on Breastfeeding & Committee on Nutrition. (2008). Prevention of rickets and vitamin D deficiency in infants, children, and adolescents. *Pediatrics, 122*(5), 1142-1152.

Wagner CL, Howard C, Hulsey TC, Lawrence RA, Taylor SN, Will H, Ebeling M, Hutson J, Hollis BW. Circulating 25-hydroxy-vitamin D Levels in Fully Breastfed Infants on Oral Vitamin D Supplementation. *J Int J Endocrin* 2010; 1-5; PCMID: 235035.

Wagner, C. L., Howard, C. R., Lawrence, R. A., Fanning, D., & Hollis, B. W. (2003). Maternal vitamin D supplementation during lactation: A viable alternative to infant supplementation. *Pediatric Research, in press*.

Wagner, C. L., Hulsey, T. C., Fanning, D., Ebeling, M., & Hollis, B.W. (2006). High Dose Vitamin D₃ Supplementation in a Cohort of Breastfeeding Mothers and Their Infants: A Six-Month Follow-up Pilot Study. *Breastfeeding Medicine, 1(2)*, 59-70.

Wagner, C. L., Johnson, D., Hulsey, T., Ebeling, M., Shary, J., Smith, P., et al. (2010a). Vitamin D supplementation during pregnancy part I NICHD/CTSA Randomized Clinical Trial (RCT): safety considerations. *Pediatric Research, in press*([abstract]).

Wagner, C. L., Taylor, S. N., & Hollis, B. W. (2008). Does vitamin D make the world go 'round'? *Breastfeeding Medicine, 3*(4), 239-250.

Wagner, C. L., Taylor, S. N., & Johnson, D. (2008). Host factors in amniotic fluid and breast milk that contribute to gut maturation. *Clinical Reviews in Allergy & Immunology, 34*(2), 191-204.

Wang, T. J., Pencina, M. J., Booth, S. L., Jacques, P. F., Ingelsson, E., Benjamin, E. J., et al. (2008). Vitamin D deficiency and risk of cardiovascular disease. *Circulation, 117*(4), 503-511.

Ward, L. (2005). Vitamin D deficiency in the 21st century: a persistent problem among Canadian infants and mothers. *CMAJ, 172*(6), 769-770.

Ward, L. M., Gaboury, I., Ladhani, M., & Zlotkin, S. (2007). Vitamin D-deficiency rickets among children in Canada. *CMAJ, 177*(2), 161-166.

Webb, A. R., deCosta, B., & Holick, M. F. (1989). Sunlight regulates the cutaneous production of vitamin D₃ by causing its photodegradation. *The Journal of Clinical Endocrinology and Metabolism, 68*, 882-887.

Webb, A. R., Kline, L., & Holick, M. F. (1988). Influence of season and latitude on the cutaneous synthesis of vitamin D₃ synthesis in human skin. *The Journal of Clinical Endocrinology and Metabolism, 67*, 373-378.

Weick, M. T. (1967). A history of rickets in the United States. *The American Journal of Clinical Nutrition, 20*(11), 1234-1241.

Weigel, N. L. (2007). Interactions between vitamin D and androgen receptor signaling in prostate cancer cells. *Nutrition Reviews, 65*(8 Pt 2), S116-117.

Weisburg, P., Scanlon, KS, Li, R, et al (2004). Nutritional rickets among children in the United States: review of cases reported between 1986 and 2003. *The American Journal of Clinical Nutrition, 80(suppl)*, 1697S-1670S.

Weishaar, R. E., Kim, S. N., Saunders, D. E., & Simpson, R. V. (1990). Involvement of vitamin D_3 with cardiovascular function III. Effects on physical and morphological properties. *The American Journal of Physiology, 258*, E134-E142.

Weishaar, R. E., & Simpson, R. V. (1987). Vitamin D_3 and cardiovascular function in rats. *The Journal of Clinical Investigation, 79*, 1706-1712.

Welch, T. R., Bergstrom, W. H., & Tsang, R. C. (2000). Vitamin D-deficient rickets: the reemergence of a once-conquered disease. *The Journal of Pediatrics, 137*(2), 143-145.

Wever, F. (1981). Absorption mechanisms for fat-soluble vitamins and the effect of other food constituents. *Progress in Clinical and Biological Research, 77*, 119.

Whiting, S., & Calvo, M. (2005). Dietary recommendations to meet both endocrine and autocrine needs of vitamin D. *The Journal of Steroid Biochemistry and Molecular Biology, 97*, 7-12.

Willer, C. J., Dyment, D. A., Sadovnick, A. D., Rothwell, P. M., Murray, T. J., & Ebers, G. C. (2005). Timing of birth and risk of multiple sclerosis: population based study. *BMJ, 330*(7483), 120.

Windaus, A., Linsert, O., Luttringhaus, A., & Weidlinch, G. (1932). Uber das krystallistierte Vitamin D_2. *Justis Liebigs Annalen der Chemie, 492*, 226-231.

Wolf, G. (2004). The discovery of vitamin D: the contribution of Adolf Windaus. *The Journal of Nutrition, 134*(6), 1299-1302.

Woolliscroft, J. (1983). Megavitamins: Fact or Fancy. *Disease-a-Month, 29*, 1-56.

Wu, K., Feskanich, D., Fuchs, C. S., Willett, W. C., Hollis, B. W., & Giovannucci, E. L. (2007). A nested case control study of plasma 25-hydroxyvitamin D concentrations and risk of colorectal cancer. *Journal of the National Cancer Institute, 99*(14), 1120-1129.

Zamora, S. A., Rizzoli, R., Belli, D. C., Slosman, D. O., & Bonjour, J. P. (1999). Vitamin D supplementaion during infancy is associated with higher bone mineral mass in prepubertal girls. *The Journal of Clinical Endocrinology and Metabolism, 84*, 4541-4543.

Zeghoud, F., Vervel, C., Guillozo, H., Walrant-Debray, O., Boutignon, H., & Garabedian, M. (1997). Subclinical vitamin D deficiency in neonates: definition and response to vitamin D supplements. *The American Journal of Clinical Nutrition, 65*(3), 771-778.

Zehnder, D., Bland, R., Williams, M., McNinch, R. W., Howie, A. J., Stewart, P., et al. (2001). Extrarenal expression of 25-hydroxyvitamin d_3-1a-hydroxylase. *The Journal of Clinical Endocrinology and Metabolism, 86*, 888-894.

Zella, L. A., Shevde, N. K., Hollis, B. W., Cooke, N. E., & Pike, J. W. (2008). Vitamin D-binding protein influences total circulating levels of 1,25-dihydroxyvitamin D_3 but does not directly modulate the bioactive levels of the hormone in vivo. *Endocrinology, 149*, 7, 3656-3667.

Zheng, Y., Niyonsaba, F., Ushio, H., Nagaoka, I., Ikeda, S., Okumura, K., et al. (2007). Cathelicidin LL-37 induces the generation of reactive oxygen species and release of human alpha-defensins from neutrophils. *British Journal of Dermatology, 157*(6), 1124-1131.

Ziegler, E. E., Hollis, B. W., Nelson, S. E., & Jeter, J. M. (2006). Vitamin D deficiency in breastfed infants in Iowa. *Pediatrics, 118*(2), 603-610.

Zittermann, A., Schleithoff, S. S., & Koerfer, R. (2005). Putting cardiovascular disease and vitamin D insufficiency into perspective. *The British Journal of Nutrition, 94*(4), 483-492.

Zittermann, A., Schleithoff, S. S., & Koerfer, R. (2006). Vitamin D insufficiency in congestive heart failure: why and what to do about it? *Heart Failure Reviews, 11*(1), 25-33.

Zittermann, A., Schleithoff, S. S., & Koerfer, R. (2007). Vitamin D and vascular calcification. *Current Opinion in Lipidology, 18*(1), 41-46.

Zittermann, A., Schleithoff, S. S., Tenderich, G., Berthold, H. K., Korfer, R., & Stehle, P. (2003). Low vitamin D status: a contributing factor in the pathogenesis of congestive heart failure? *Journal of the American College of Cardiology, 41*(1), 105-112.

INDEX

E

F

G

H

I

L

M

N

O

P

R

S

T

AUTHOR BIOS

Dr. Carol Wagner, a board-certified pediatrician and neonatologist, has extensive experience in clinical studies. She is an attending neonatologist and Professor of Pediatrics at the Medical University of South Carolina (MUSC). She has been a member of ISRHML since 1995, a member of the American Academy of Pediatrics' Breastfeeding and Perinatal sections, a Fellow in the Academy of Breastfeeding Medicine, and is an elected member in the 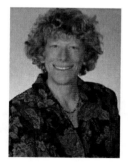 Society for Pediatric Research and the American Society for Nutritional Sciences. Her clinical activities as a neonatologist dovetail with her strong research interests in human milk, lactation, and vitamin D. Dr. Wagner has written several articles about breastfeeding, growth factors and structure in human milk, and vitamin D requirements in pregnant and lactating women. She is co-principal investigator with Dr. Bruce Hollis of a recently completed NIH/NICHD-supported vitamin D supplementation trial involving pregnant women and their infants and an ongoing clinical trial of vitamin D supplementation involving lactating women and their infants. She is also principal investigator of another recently completed trial funded by the Thrasher Research Fund involving vitamin D supplementation of pregnant women in community health centers, with ongoing three-year follow-up of the children. Dr. Wagner actively collaborates with Drs. Hollis and Taylor on several ongoing vitamin D and human milk studies.

Dr. Sarah Taylor is a board-certified pediatrician and neonatologist, and as an academic clinician is involved in vitamin D research. She performed her residency in Pediatrics and fellowship in Neonatal-Perinatal Medicine at MUSC in Charleston, South Carolina, after completing medical school at the University Of Miami Miller School Of Medicine. Dr. Taylor joined the MUSC Division of Neonatology in 2005. Her research interest is preterm 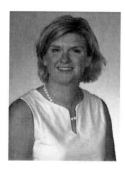 infant nutrition and growth, with special emphasis on breastmilk and vitamin

D. She currently is conducting an NIH-funded study of the vitamin D needs of preterm infants and collaborates with Drs. Wagner and Hollis on several related vitamin D studies.

Dr. Bruce Hollis is one of the world's leading experts on vitamin D and calcium homeostasis, with more than three decades of active research in the field. He received his undergraduate and master's degrees in Science from Ohio State University and his Ph.D. from University of Guelph, Ontario, Canada. He is a tenured professor at the Medical University of South Carolina, where he has worked since 1986. He has personally developed many of the laboratory 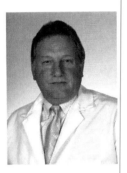 assays in use in the world today. Dr. Hollis holds the first Investigational New Drug number issued by the FDA in the study of high dose vitamin D supplementation during pregnancy. He is the principal investigator of the recently completed NIH/NICHD vitamin D randomized control trial during pregnancy and of the ongoing NIH/NICHD vitamin D randomized control trial during lactation. He serves on the board of D-Action Grassroots Health and is an international leader in the field of vitamin D research. Dr. Hollis actively collaborates with Drs. Wagner and Taylor on several ongoing vitamin D projects.

Ordering Information

Hale Publishing, L.P.

1712 N. Forest Street

Amarillo, Texas, USA 79106

8:00 am to 5:00 pm CST

Call » 806.376.9900

Sales » 800.378.1317

Fax » 806.376.9901

Online Web Orders

www.ibreastfeeding.com